FLOSSING

A CIP record for this book is available from the British Library

ISBN 978-1-85097-296-9

Publisher's address
Quintessence Publishing Co, Ltd
Quintessence House
Grafton Road, New Malden, Surrey KT3 3AB
United Kingdom

Address for correspondence/authors' contact details
Roland Kreutzer: r.kreutzer@gmx.de
Klaas Stechmann: info@fdm-therapeut.de
Hendrik Eggers: Hendrik.Eggers@hotmail.de
Bernard C. Kolster: berndkolster@me.com

QUINTESSENCE PUBLISHING

www.quintpub.co.uk

1st edition, 2016

Translation: Rosana Jelaska, Lymington/UK
Copy editor: Markus Polzer, Berlin
Photographs: Martin Kreutter, Marburg
Layout and typesetting: David Kühn, Berlin
Cover design: David Kühn, Berlin
Overall production: Quintessenz Verlags-GmbH, Berlin
Printed by: Grafički zavod Hrvatske, Zagreb

Printed in Croatia

Important information

Like every other science, medicine is constantly evolving. Research and clinical experience widen our knowledge. If any treatment recommendations are mentioned in this book, the reader may have confidence that the authors, editor, and publisher have taken great care to ensure that this information is in line with the latest knowledge available at the time of publication. However, the publisher cannot give guarantees for any information regarding the forms, techniques, and frequencies of treatment application. Every treatment takes place at the user's own responsibility.

FLOSSING

ROLAND KREUTZER

KLAAS STECHMANN

HENDRIK EGGERS

BERNARD C. KOLSTER (ED.)

The authors (f. l. t. r.)

Hendrik Eggers is a physiotherapist (B. Sc.) in Lüneburg. For some time now, he has been concentrating his attention on flossing and its practical applications.

Roland Kreutzer is an instructor in the Brügger approach for the management of musculoskeletal disorders and a manual therapist. He has 25 years of practical experience concerning disorders in the areas of orthopedic medicine, surgery, and pediatric orthopedics. He regularly gives courses to pass on his knowledge and his wealth of experience.

Klaas Stechmann is a physiotherapist, naturopath, and master's degree student in osteopathy. He is an independent practitioner at interdisciplinary group practices in Hamburg and Stade. For over five years, the focus of his work has been on the fascia system and its significance to the human body.

Dr. Bernard C. Kolster (ed.) is a physiotherapist and physician. His main areas of practice are physical medicine, rehabilitation, reflex therapy, and nutritional medicine. He is author and editor of many specialist textbooks.

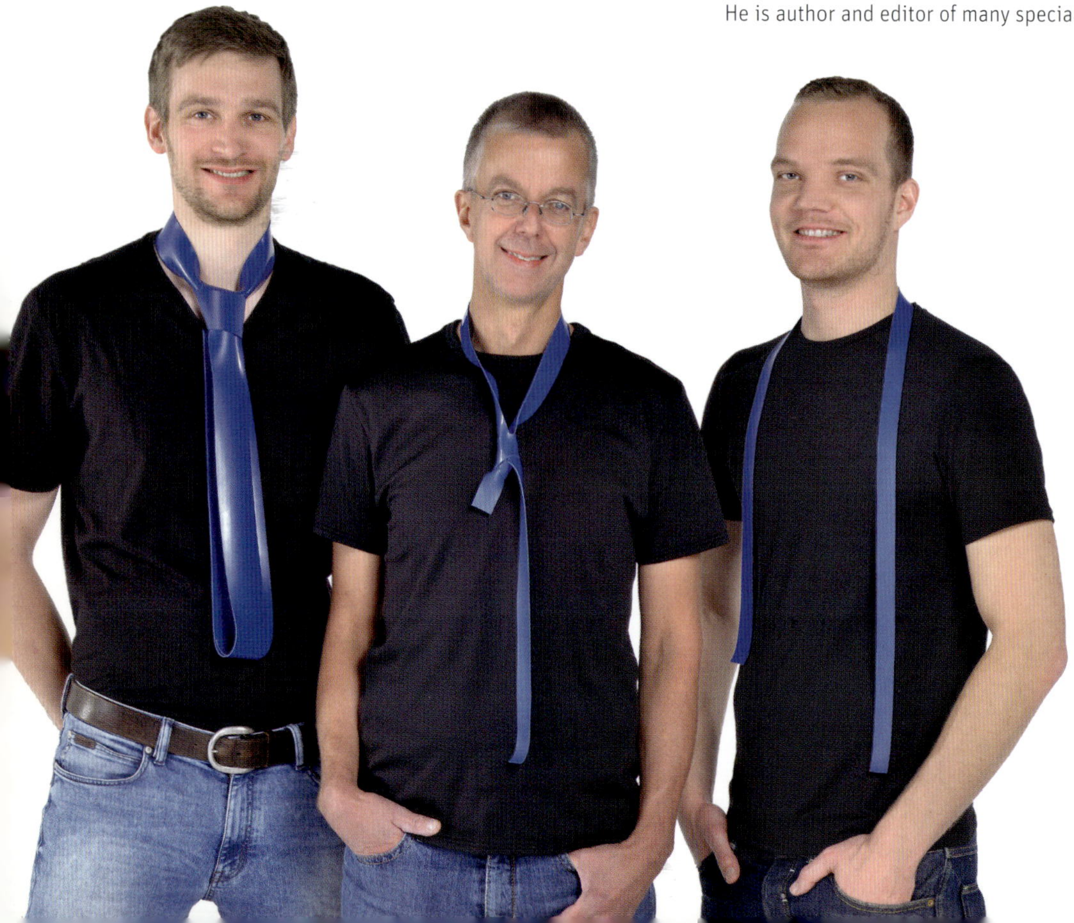

Foreword

Dear Readers,

in recent times, there has been a lot of hype on the subject of "flossing". However, the available study evidence in this area is still sparse. Before the launch of this book, there was previously just one (!) German-language article (Seidenspinner & Kolster 2015). It was therefore high time to pay closer attention to this form of therapy. The conclusion was this: the way that flossing band treatments work appears not only perplexing, but even somewhat mystical.

Our many years of joint physiotherapeutic experience in this subject area form the foundation for this guide – the world's first – which provides a comprehensive description of the basic principles and potential applications of flossing. We have designed this work for therapists and athletes, to allow common pain syndromes and the typical injuries sustained in a variety of sports to be treated effectively with flossing wraps, as an adjunct to previously available therapeutic options. A further, important plus point of flossing for the treatment of pain is that the body suffers no added exposure to medication, so that the technique can be used in many patient groups, provided that any contraindications that exist are observed. What can be achieved with flossing? Typical pain, such as that caused by muscle tightness, inflamed tendons, painful joints, or swellings, can be treated effectively with the flossing band. In addition, flossing can also be used specifically for muscle-building and strength sports. This is backed up by sound studies and investigations.

Flossing is by no means a stand-alone method. The description of each of the flossing wraps depicted here is preceded by an exploration of the causes of the pain syndromes and sports injuries in question. After this, the wrap is explained step by step and illustrated with a series of photographs. Active exercises to be performed by the user with the flossing band in place are shown at the end of each section.

This book contains two parts: the first part conveys the theoretical basics as regards mechanism of action, applied tension, and the possibilities and limitations of the method. Various application techniques are also explained with the aid of examples. The practical part that follows presents potential applications on individual regions and structures of the body. Logically structured series of images and clear explanations introduce the user to "flossing", step by step.

As already mentioned at the beginning, flossing is an experience-based therapy form which is yet to be subjected to rigorous scientific testing. With this work, the authors would like to document the current state of knowledge and encourage all therapists to involve themselves actively in the further development of flossing.

Last but not least, at this point we want to thank all of those involved who contributed to the creation of this book: David Kühn of KVM-Verlag must take the lead here. Without his stringent project management and his creativity in realizing the text and illustrations, this book would never have come about with such high quality, and certainly not at such breathtaking speed. Thankfully, our copy editor of the first German edition Renate Mannaa was able to keep up with that tempo, even if she repeatedly had to drop everything else in favor of this project. Thank you, Ms. Mannaa! Furthermore, we would to thank Rosana Jelaska for her outstanding English translation of the book. A big, big thank you also goes to our awesome model Martin, with his patience and apparent immunity to pain and to our photographer Martin Kreutter for his excellent work behind the camera and for providing us with such outstanding images.

We wish all our readers and therapists, all users of flossing, new or experienced, rewarding treatment and training results with flossing band wraps, and we hope that our book can play a part in achieving this. We look forward to your feedback!

The authors, September 2016

Roland Kreutzer
Klaas Stechmann
Hendrik Eggers
Bernard C. Kolster (ed.)

Table of contents

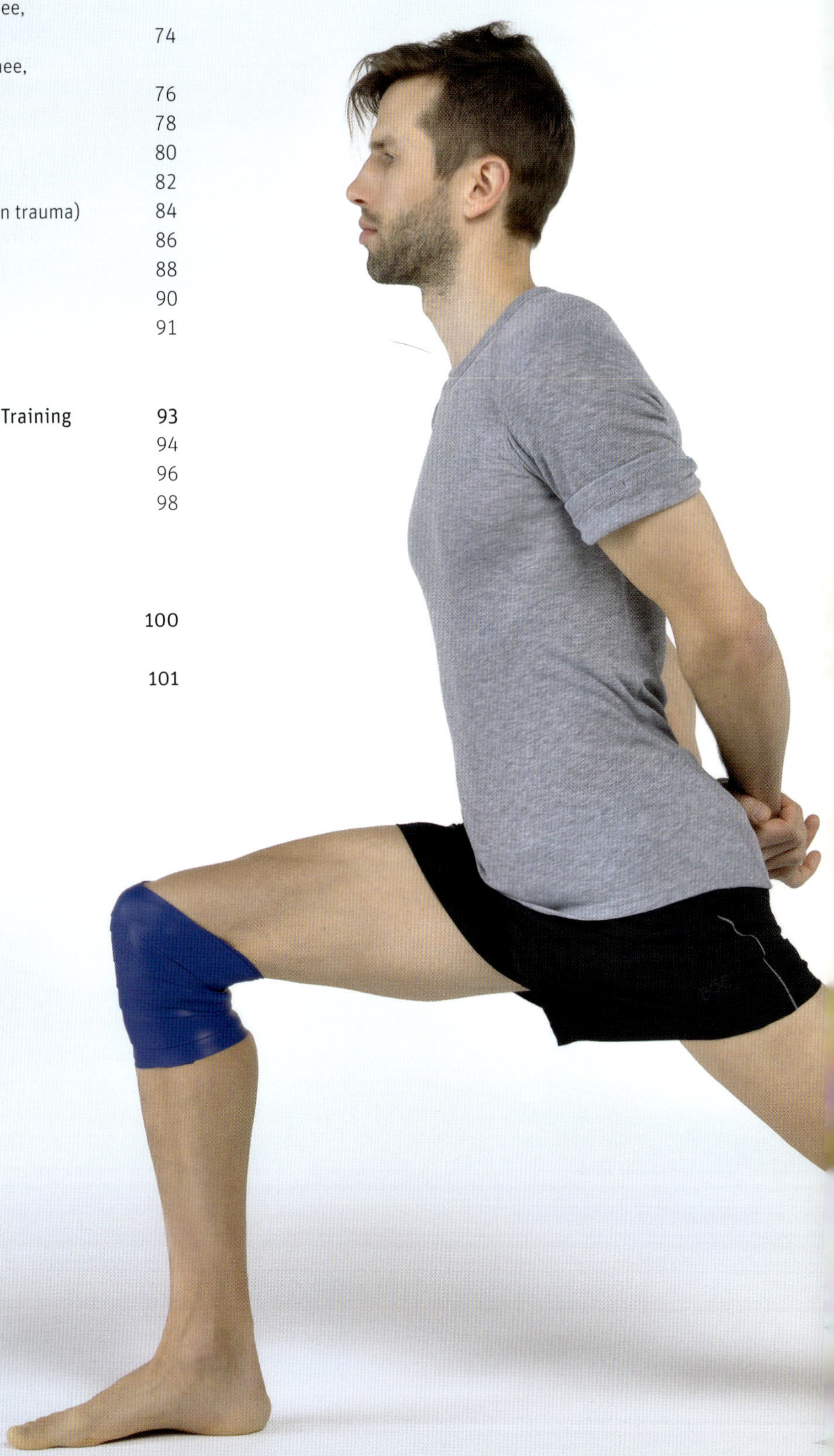

Flossing –
The Basics

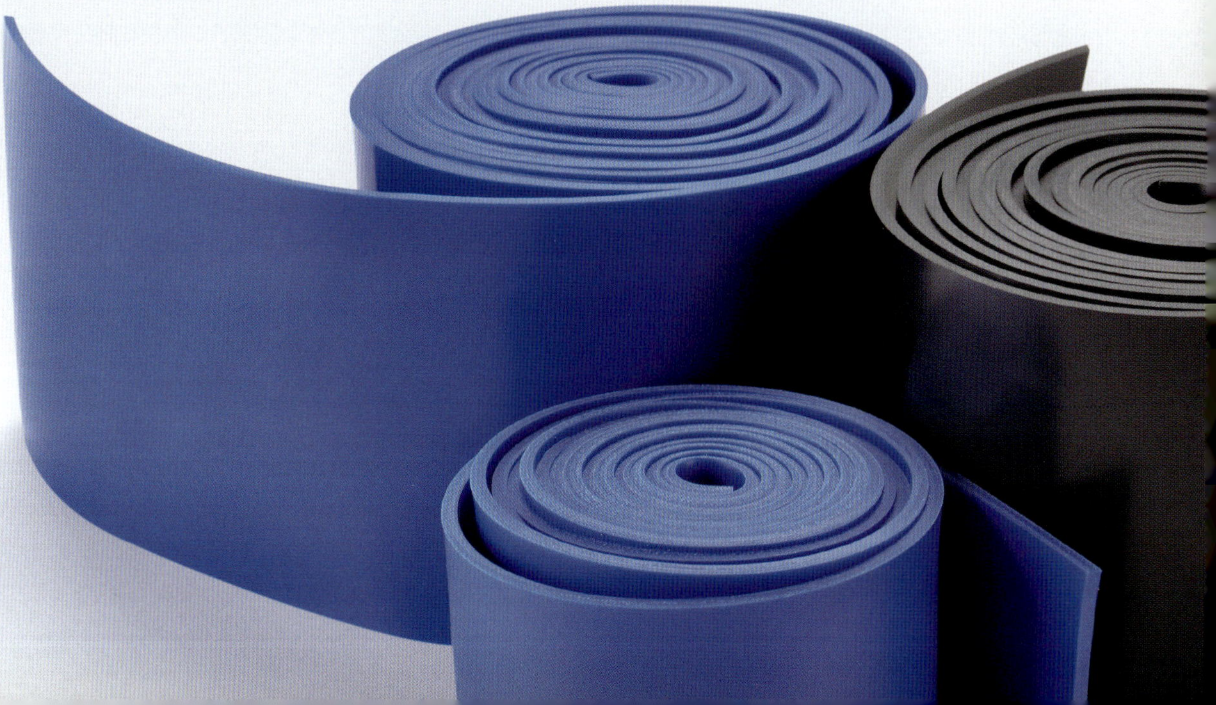

What is flossing?

In everyday usage, the words "floss" and "flossing" refer to the use of dental floss in oral and dental hygiene. More recently, in a worldwide trend, "flossing" has acquired a new meaning, namely the specific use of elastic bands in the areas of training and rehabilitation. This involves compression bandages made of elastic rubber bands, which are applied to treat disorders of the musculoskeletal system.
The method has often been referred to as "voodoo flossing" due to its astonishingly good effect, which could not be explained with any degree of certainty (in this context, "voodoo" may be interpreted to mean an obscure, unexplainable witchcraft).

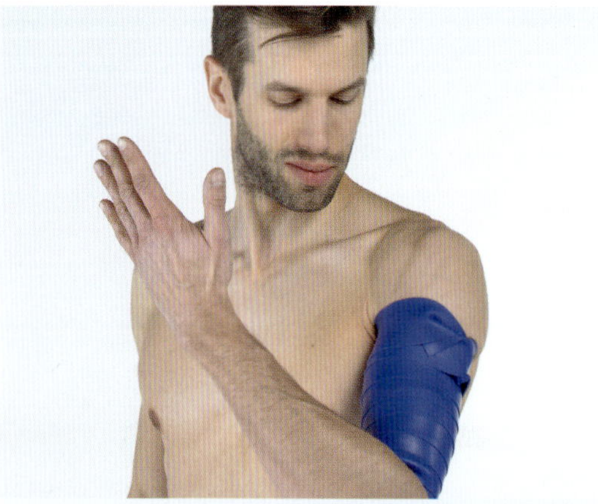

The clear aims of flossing

- Pain relief
- Improved mobility
- Reduction of swellings
- Building and strengthening muscle
- Improved coordination

Recently, it was Kelly Starrett who included the term "voodoo flossing" and the treatment method itself in his book on fitness training (Starrett 2014).

The elastic bands are wound directly around the extremity affected by pain, restricted mobility and acute swellings, and the extremity is then actively moved. The treatment's aims are pain relief, improved mobility, the reduction of swellings, and rapid healing. Increased use of the method in medical training therapy has now also paved the way for hypotheses to explain its efficacy.

Material

Flossing bands (see Fig. 1) are made of 100% natural rubber and are available in various lengths of approx. 1.03 to 2.06 m. The thickness of the material varies between 1.1 mm and 1.6 mm. Bands used on arms, legs, and the body are 5 cm wide. Shorter and narrower bands 2.5 cm in width are available for use on small joints and the hands. Apart from correct technique, the quality of the bands is a key factor for a successful treatment. The surface of the band must not be too smooth, i.e. it needs to show the necessary grip. Elasticity plays another important role.

The band has to fit well and cling to the skin to the optimal extent. Only good elasticity and fit can lead to the desired therapeutic stimulus in the tissues and target structures. The uniform elasticity allows the tension to be dosed accurately and adjusted individually to the structures being manipulated. Flossing bands are free of softeners and other toxic substances and are therefore safe for use on the skin. However, an allergy to rubber will need to be ruled out beforehand. If such an allergy is present, the flossing band may be applied over clothing.

How to recognice a "good" band for use in flossing

A suitable band has a very slightly silky surface; it must not feel smooth. When the band is pulled, its resistance should be soft but elastic, and the band should stretch uniformly. Regardless of the brand or manufacturer you choose, make sure that the surface and elastic stretch are as described.

Material properties

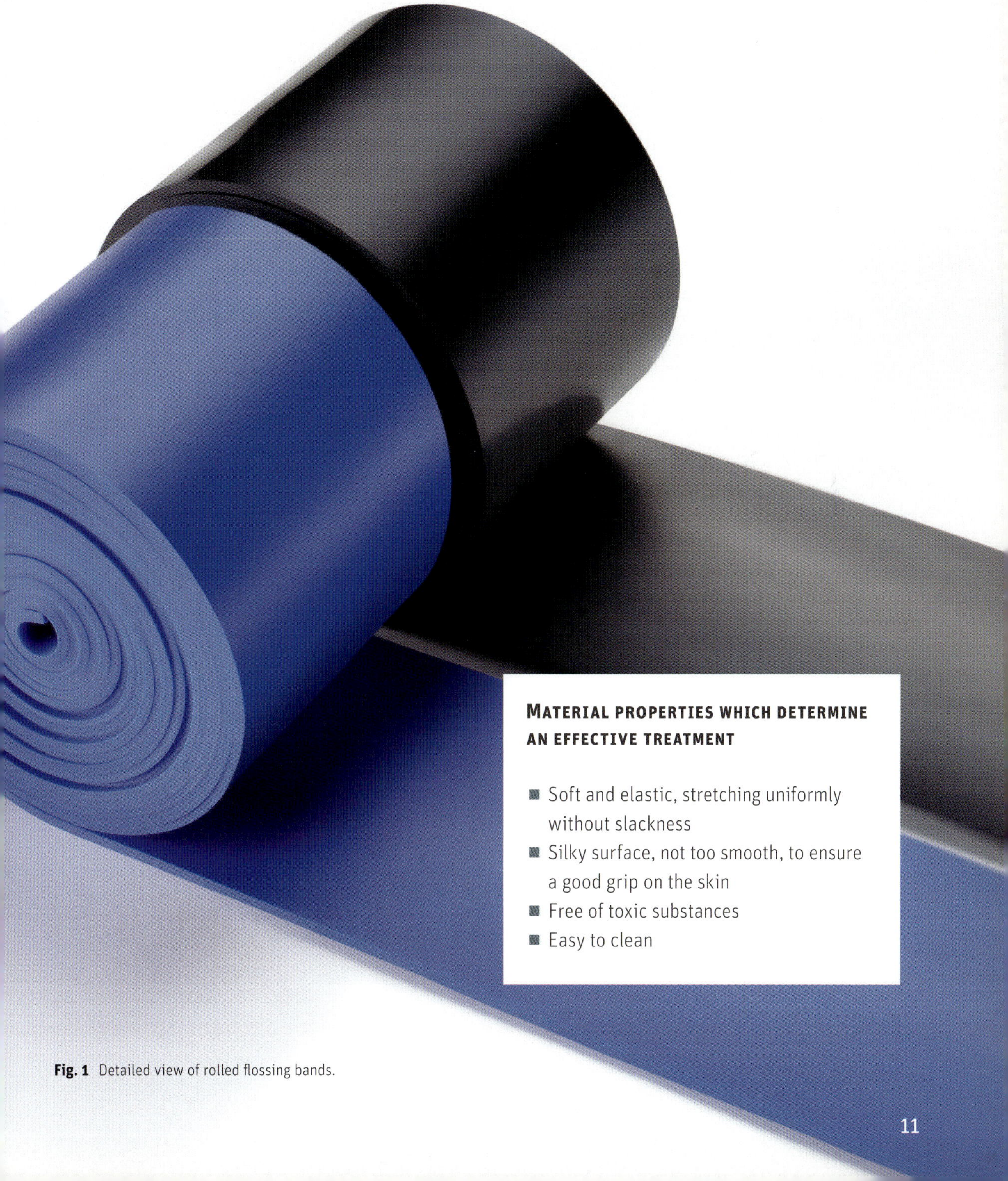

MATERIAL PROPERTIES WHICH DETERMINE AN EFFECTIVE TREATMENT

- Soft and elastic, stretching uniformly without slackness
- Silky surface, not too smooth, to ensure a good grip on the skin
- Free of toxic substances
- Easy to clean

Fig. 1 Detailed view of rolled flossing bands.

Mechanisms of action

Blood flow and tissue drainage

To date, there are only very few scientific studies on flossing. Its exact active principle has not been clearly elucidated as yet, although there are a number of possible effects. The mechanism of action of flossing bands is not attributed exclusively to their compression, since additional movements always need to be performed.

When the band is tightly wound, this immediately reduces blood flow in the treatment area. Tissue fluid is squeezed out by the elastic ligature (see Fig. 2). The subsequent rapid loosening of the ligature leads to immediate, enhanced blood flow, which one might picture as a sponge effect (see Fig. 3). Metabolic by-products are pretty much squeezed out by the compression and are then washed out by the subsequent hyperemia. In general, the compression is released again after 1–2 minutes, immediately allowing blood and lymph to circulate freely again.

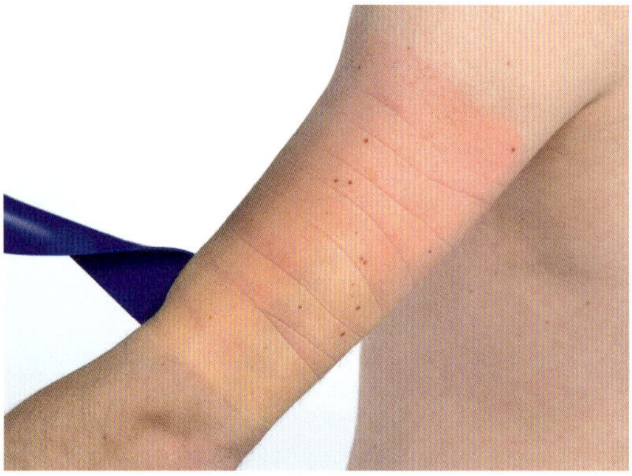

Fig. 2 The blood is forced out by the powerful compression.

At the level of the lymphatic system, one might imagine that the powerful pressure transports swellings into regions with a functioning lymphatic system. Recent studies show that optimal pressures for the reduction of edema can be considerably higher than previously recommended in lymphatic drainage (Taradaj et al. 2015; Zaleska et al. 2014). Thus, pressures of around 120 mmHg (equivalent to 0.16 kg/cm^2) show the best edema reduction when the transient compression is repeated several times. For now, the mechanisms of action of lymphatic drainage in flossing remain a matter for speculation, because no studies on the subject currently exist.

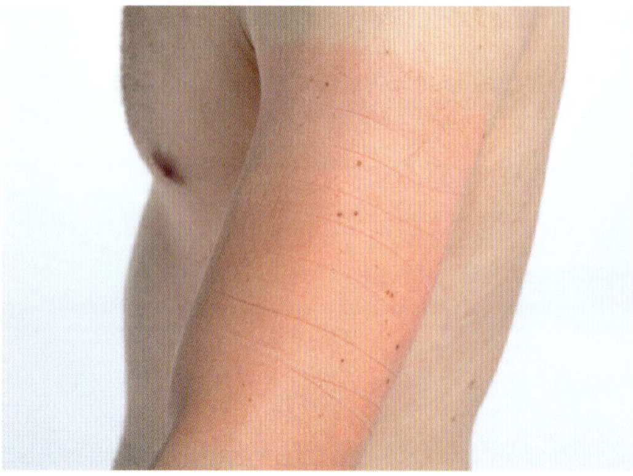

Fig. 3 The diminished blood flow is immediately followed by intense reddening of the treated area.

Skin and fascia network

The skin is in direct contact with the flossing band and conducts the stimuli to the central nervous system via numerous receptors (see Fig. 4). The intensive flossing treatment of the skin leads to powerful stimulation of the mechanoreceptors and the conduction of these stimuli to the brain causes suppression of pain stimuli in the spinal cord. This increased input also enables the nervous system to compensate for any discrepancies and imbalances.

The body's fascial network begins directly below the skin. Thanks to the fact that they are prolifically supplied with nerve fibers and receptors, and to their ability to bind water, fascias may be defined as the body's biggest sensory organ. The fascial network links all the body's organs, from head to foot and from the outside in. The central element is the mobility of the individual fascia layers and their relationship with neighboring structures such as tendons, muscles, ligaments, blood vessels, and nerve fibers (see Fig. 5).

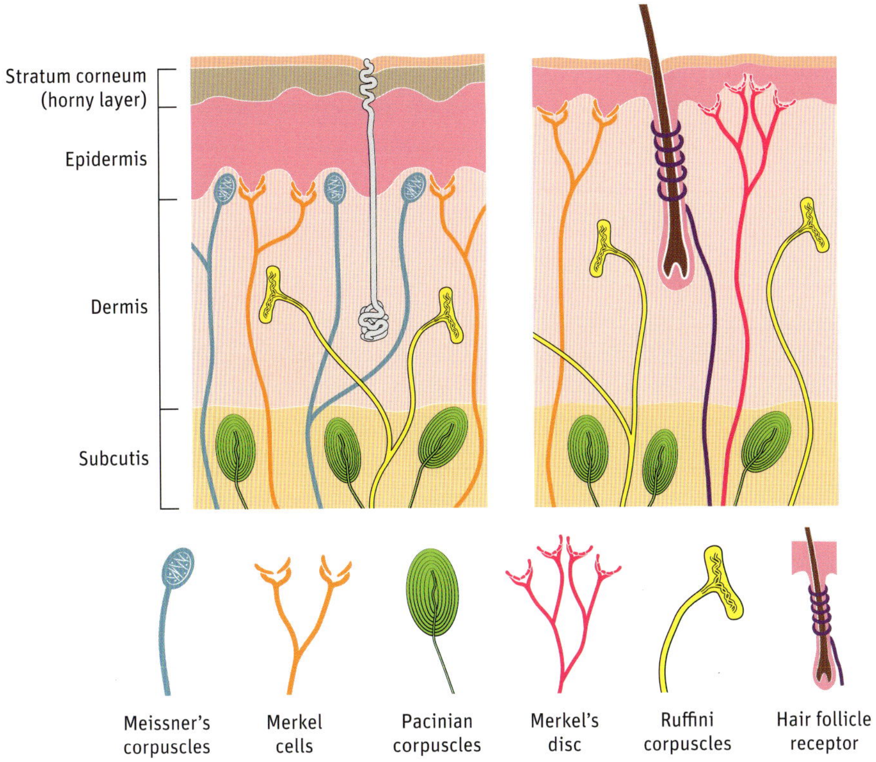

Fig. 4 The numerous mechanoreceptors of the skin and fascia conduct the therapeutic stimulus to the spinal cord and brain.

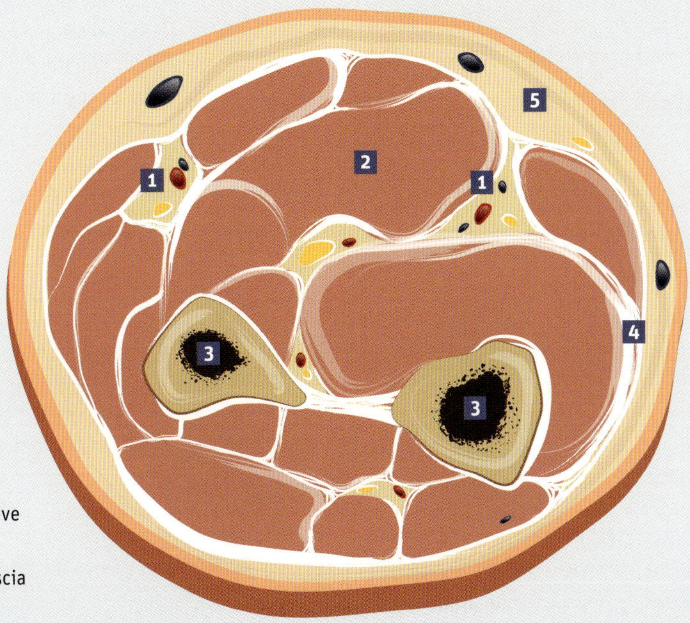

1 Veins, nerves, and arteries
2 Musculature
3 Bone
4 Intermuscular connective tissue and fascias
5 Skin and superficial fascia of the body

Fig. 5 Forearm in cross-section. The relative positions of bone, muscles, fascias, blood vessels, and nerves are clearly visible. On compression by the flossing band and simultaneous movement of the arm, the resultant shear forces cause mobilization of the various levels.

Injuries, surgery, and insufficient exercise can lead to adhesions, and thus also to impairments in the fascia. If flossing is seen as a treatment for the fascia, it is easy to explain why flossing is particularly effective following surgery and injuries. The pressure of the band, combined with the concomitant movement, generates shear forces. The individual layers are held in place from the outside, whereas the active movement taking place at the same time loosens adhesions between the individual layers (see Fig. 6).

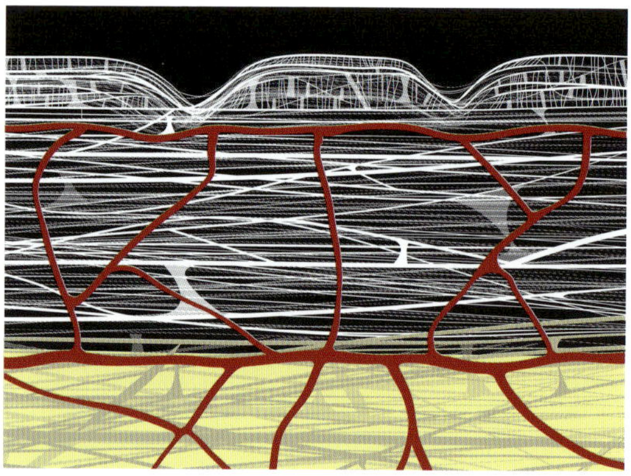

Fig. 6 This image illustrates the continuity of the collagen fibers from the skin's surface to the deeper layers. The sliding movements take place in these regions. Blood vessels (red) and other structures such as tendons and nerve fibers need to be able to move freely (modified from Guimberteau 2015).

Furthermore, compression and stimulation of the mechanoreceptors demonstrably leads to an improved fluid supply to the extracellular matrix ("ground substance") (Schleip 2003). The increased water content reduces viscosity and, in turn, results in increased mobility. The outstanding efficacy of flossing in patients who have undergone surgery in the more distant past can be explained by the restoration of fascial mobility. Similarly, persistent long-term effects are presumably associated with restored fascial integrity.

Joints

If a joint is included in the wrap, perceptible compression of that entire joint takes place. The joint capsules and surrounding ligaments contain proprioceptors, which provide the brain and the vestibular system with information about the positions of the joints and the stresses to which they are subjected. Joint effusion frequently occurs due to a joint injury – distortion/sprain – or following surgery, causing pain and restricted mobility of the joint capsule. This inhibits both coordination and the sensorimotor functions. The astonishing effect of flossing can certainly trigger proprioceptive/sensorimotor reintegration. Accelerated response times in the treated muscles have been seen in EMG studies (Seidenspinner & Kolster 2015).

NOTE

To achieve the maximum possible effect, the flossing band should be applied directly to the skin.

This could explain the immediate effects that take place. The direction of the band's pull can be used to exert a specific stimulus on the position of the joint. Thus, winding the band with the direction of pull from the inside out brings about a slight lateral displacement of the moving parts of the joint (see Fig. 7). As a result, the movement causes distraction of certain segments of the joint. Occasionally, this results in release of the joint, with an audible crack during the flossing movement.

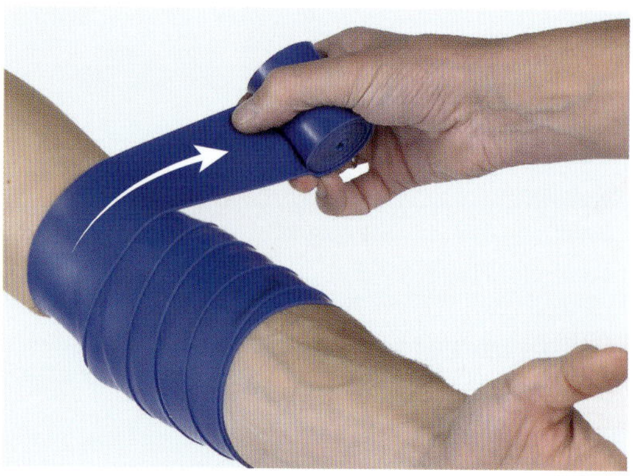

Fig. 7 In tennis elbow, the band is wound with increasing tension from the inside out. This may cause a slight lateral distraction effect.

Biochemical factors

The consequence of movement with a reduced blood supply is that the blood collects in the bound area. The muscle fatigues considerably more quickly. Oxygen saturation and pH decrease as a result. Thus, there is more rapid accumulation of lactic acid which eventually leads to an increased release of growth hormones (Fig. 8). The muscle cells also swell. These are effects similar to those seen following intensive maximum strength training with heavy weights.

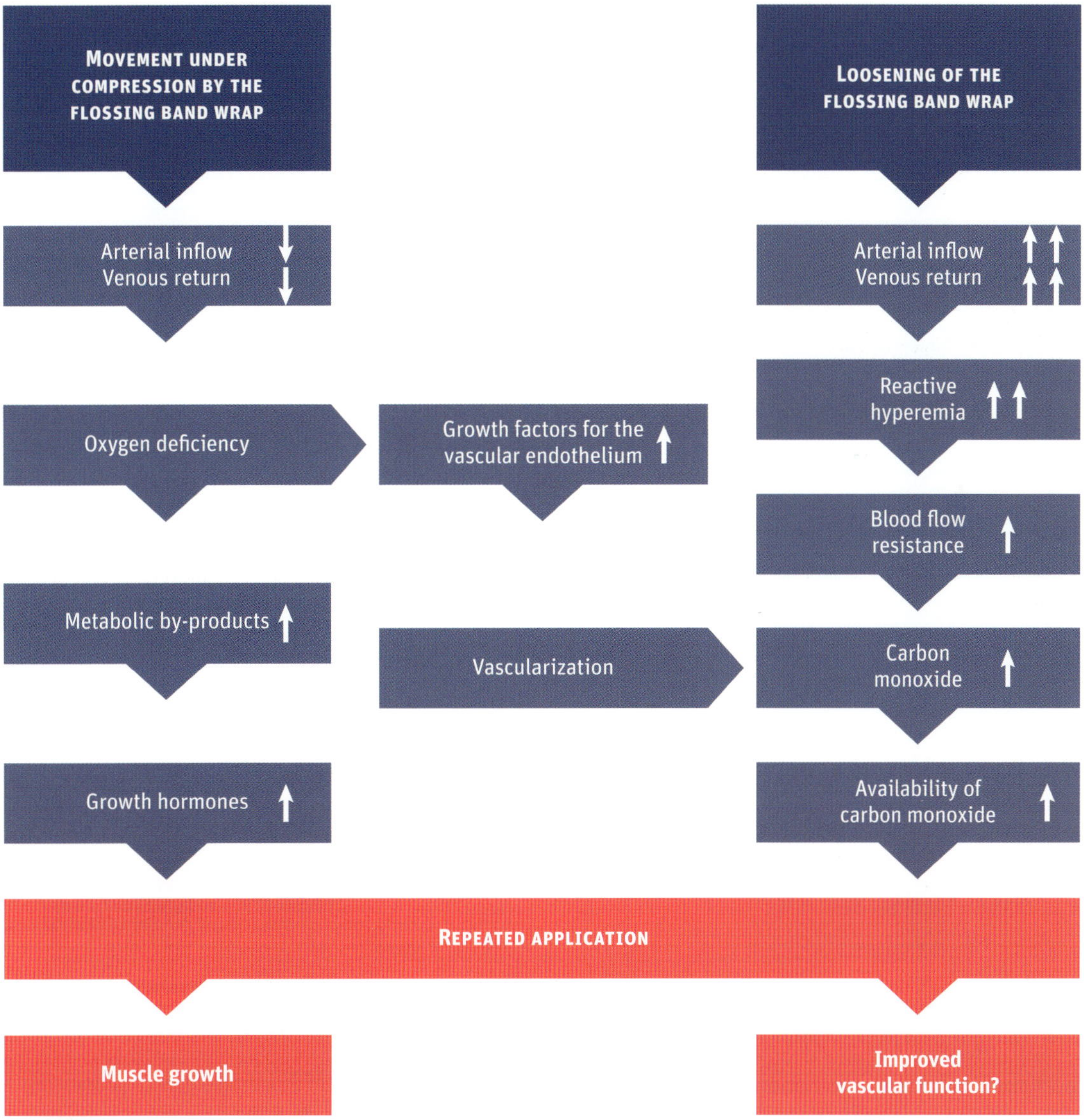

Fig. 8 Flow chart of the processes which occur under blood stasis due to compression with simultaneous training, modified from Horiuchi & Okita 2012 *(? = There is as yet no clear evidence for the relevant changes.)*

Mechanisms of action

Pain and endogenous inhibition

Pain needs to be taken seriously as a therapeutic mechanism of action. If a painful stimulus is applied, processes referred to as descending inhibition are initiated in the brain, spinal cord, and nerve fibers. Pain is blocked by the endogenous release of opioids and healing stimuli. In simplified terms, this course of events may be interpreted as stimulation of the body's self-healing powers. The efficacy of the frequently underestimated placebo effect is also better if therapeutic stimuli are more intensely perceived.

PLAUSIBLE MECHANISMS OF ACTION – A SUMMARY:

- "Sponge" or irrigation effect at the cellular level
  - *Squeezing out the tissue by compression*
  - *Saturation or "flushing" due to abrupt hyperemia*
  - *Lymphatic drainage as a result of the applied pressure*
- At tissue level
  - *Shear effects which lead to mobilization of various structures – skin, fascias, muscles, tendons, joint capsules, neural structures, setc.*
  - *Reduced viscosity of the extracellular matrix*
- Decongestion of joint effusions, with a resultant increase in the range of motion
- Direct influence on proprioception and sensorimotor function in the form of proprioceptive or sensorimotor reintegration as a result of forced movement under compression
- Decreasing pain inhibition due to the intensive treatment stimulus
- Biochemical factors
  - *Change in the metabolic situation*
  - *Accumulation of lactate*
  - *pH reduction*
  - *Release of growth hormones*

Areas of use

In general, flossing is used to treat pain and restricted mobility of the extremities and trunk:

- Muscle pain
- Pain and restricted mobility of the ligaments and joints
- Swellings
- Localized, stabbing pain
- Postoperative scars and adhesions
- For muscle-building (blood flow restriction training or occlusion training)
- For regeneration after training, for muscle soreness
- Could also be useful for spasticity and painful hemiparesis, perhaps with the aid of passive movement

Flossing is particularly relevant in the following conditions:

- Pain and injuries of the shoulder and upper arm
- Following shoulder surgery
- Tennis elbow
- Golfer's elbow
- Pain in the wrists, finger joints, also the metacarpophalangeal and first carpometacarpal joints of the thumb
- Carpal tunnel syndrome
- (Acute) swellings of the arm
- Problems in the thoracic spine and ribs (e.g. when breathing)
- Pain and restricted movement in the lumbar spine as well as the sacroiliac joints (SIJ) and symphysis

How to use flossing

- Pain in the knee joints, also including the patellar tendon, the ligaments and the menisci
- Following surgery to the lower extremity, especially the knee
- Pain and inflammation of the calf muscles and Achilles tendon
- Pain and swellings of the ankle joint
- Supination trauma
- Pain due to heel spur, plantar fasciitis and hallux valgus, pain in the toe joints

Contraindications

Use on the skin is conditional on the absence of open wounds or severe skin irritation. Flossing should not be undertaken if the following conditions or restrictions are present:

- Injuries and burns in the affected area
- Rubber allergy, although application over clothing may be possible
- Acute inflammation caused by microbial infection
- Thromboses and acute venous disorders
- Arterial occlusive disease
- Cancerous tumors, as there is a risk of metastasization
- Refusal of the treatment
- Chronic heart failure, due to the risk of volume overload
- Chronic inflammatory disorder such as gout: overheating, reddening, swelling, pain, functional impairment
- The use of oral agent that inhibit blood clotting: anticoagulants and new antiplatelet drugs

Relative contraindication (use with caution)

- Psychological components: the patient feels unpleasantly restricted by the bandaging.

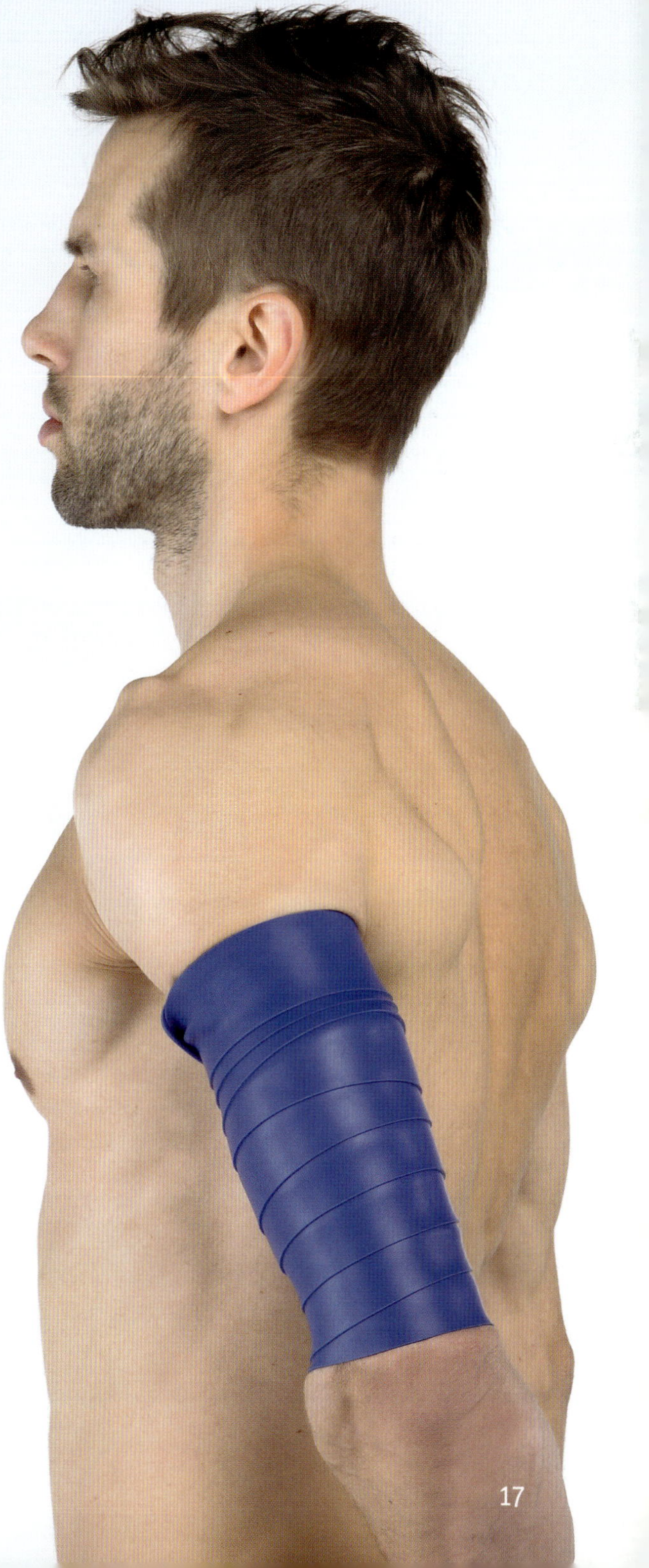

How to use flossing

After-effects and side effects

Since flossing works with a very powerful stimulus, there may be some side effects:

- Hematomas: the patient should be informed about this, as hematomas should be regarded as a physical injury (see Fig. 9)
- Skin pain: after the treatment, this may be treated with the "smoothing" technique (see Fig. 16, p. 21).
- Short-term faintness
- Vegetative symptoms: circulatory insufficiency, outbreaks of sweating

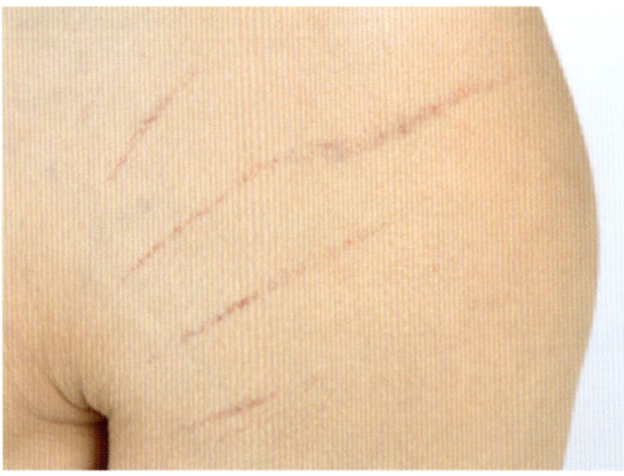

Fig. 9 In some cases, flossing treatments may lead to hematomas. These are harmless, but the patient should be informed about this before the treatment.

Cleaning/disinfection and care of the flossing band

It is advisable for every patient to possess his or her own flossing band – for self-treatment and for hygiene reasons. After contact with the skin, the band should be cleaned under running water and then dried. Disinfection with commonly available agents for the sterilization of materials is also possible.

Practical application of the band

As a general rule, the bands are applied very tightly. The treatment is usually painful, but should still be tolerable. Familiarize yourself and the person undergoing flossing with the band and the procedure. If progressive tingling or very severe pain occur during the treatment, the band must be removed without delay.

Patient information

The patient should be informed about the significance and purpose of the treatment, and also about the potential side effects and accessory phenomena, such as bruises. The following subjects should form part of this information:

- Pain reduction
- Improving the range of motion
- Loosening adhesions
- Improved circulation
- Painfulness of the treatment
- Possible bruising
- The treatment can be stopped at any time
- No severe pain should occur below the wrap
- It is essential for the patient to communicate any discomfort, pain, and numbness

Tension

Flossing is most effectively used if the direction of pull and the applied tension are utilized in targeted fashion to increase the therapeutic effect. The tension determines the strength of the compression and thus also the intensity of the therapeutic stimulus. In principle, the band should be wound with 50% tension at the first turn; as wrapping proceeds, the applied tension is increased to 60–80%. Test the stretch of the band in advance to get a feel for the level of tension (see Fig. 10).

The rule of thumb is to increase the applied tension further at the problem site. Swellings are generally treated with only 50% tension and uniform pressure.

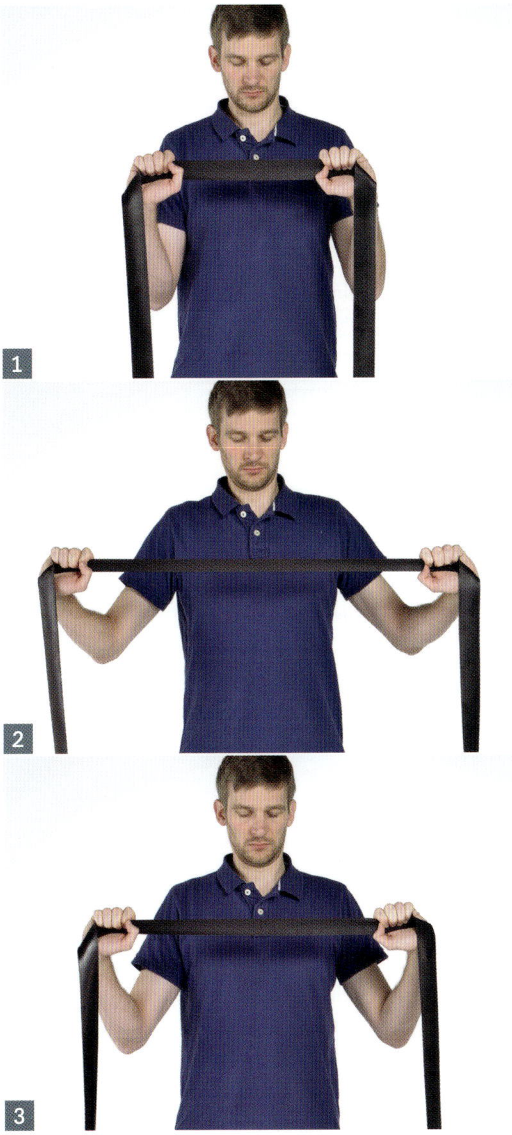

Fig. 10 The flossing band in neutral position with no pull (1). Pull the band apart to maximum stretch; this corresponds to 100% tension (2). A tension of approximately 60–80% is equivalent to treatment intensity (3).

Direction of pull and direction of effect

The direction in which the band is applied also determines the direction of its effect. Always wrap the band in ascending turns relative to the body, to ensure better transport away from the treatment site. In principle, the band should be applied with up to 50% overlap at each turn (see Fig. 11). The direction of pull can be used specifically to intensify effects on a joint.

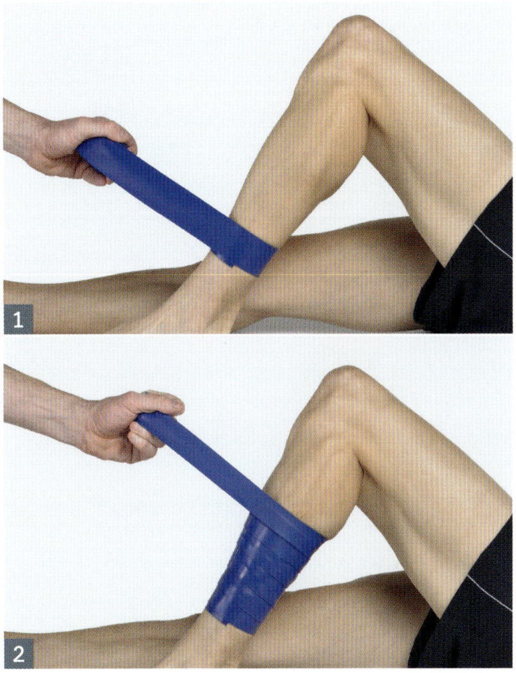

Fig. 11 The first turn is applied with about 50% tension (1). The band is then wrapped with ascending turns at an increased pull of 60–80%, with around 50% overlap at each turn (2).

APPLYING AND WRAPPING THE BAND

- Wrap with ascending turns
- Start with 50% tension
- When wrapping the affected area, increase the applied tension to 60–80%
- The band overlaps around 50% at each ascending turn
- Perform movements to the maximum extent possible and with varying levels of resistance
- Remove the band after around 2 minutes

Where to use flossing

Application site

The nature and method of application are determined by the symptoms. For example, if the upper arm is flossed to treat biceps muscle problems, the pull should be increased on the anterior side, i.e. over the affected area. Should one wish to apply intense compression to a joint, the entire joint should be included in the wrap. Conversely, if the focus is on the surrounding muscles, the joint may be left out, and the band wound more tightly above and below it. It is also possible to apply additional turns, perhaps crossing the band over at the site of the most severe symptoms (see Fig. 12).

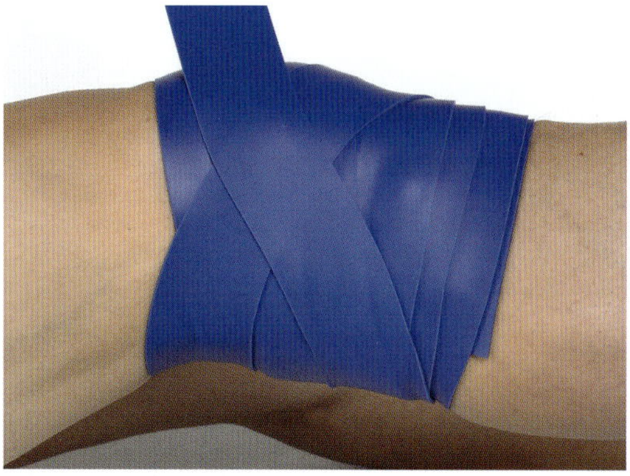

Fig. 12 Applying an additional crossover turn can intensify the therapeutic effect.

The movements

Nach der Wickelung sind die ausgeführten Bewegungen The movements performed after the band is applied are the most important factor of the treatment. These movements should start slowly, but should extend rapidly over the full range of motion of the area being treated. The movement that is performed needs to be guided by the painful movements hitherto experienced by the patient. If the person being treated cannot execute the movement to its fullest range, some passive assistance may be given. Functional movements which affect several joints are also a good idea. The effect can be intensified with the use of weights or resistance exercises. For example, if pain occurs during strength training, and flossing without weight-bearing can no longer produce an improvement, the exercise should be carried out with more resistance, rather like functional training (see Fig. 13).

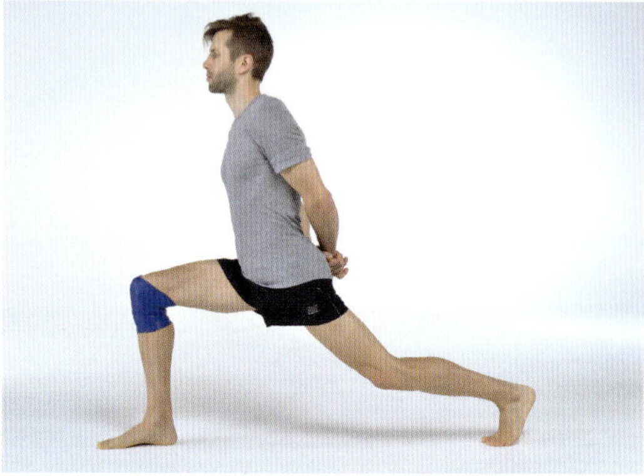

Fig. 13 As far as possible, the movements should be performed in a number of variants and over the full range of motion. Lunges are one example of a functional movement.

Checking blood flow

During the treatment, the blood supply can be checked by feeling the pulse at the wrist, the back of the foot or the inner side of the ankle (see Fig. 14).

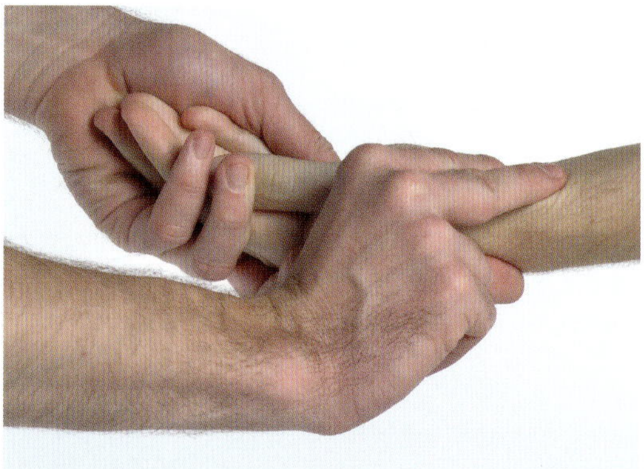

Fig. 14 Checking blood flow by feeling the pulse on the inside of the wrist.

General treatment tips

Another way of checking blood flow is to apply pressure with the fingers to see whether the test area goes red again when the pressure is released, rather than staying white (see Fig. 15).

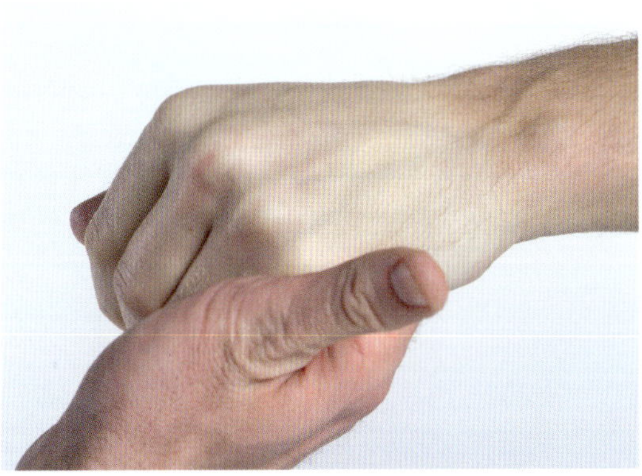

Fig. 15 Checking blood flow by testing reactive reddening of the skin after applying pressure with the fingers.

FACTORS WHICH INFLUENCE FLOSSING

- Direction of pull and applied tension
- Application site
- The movement performed when the band is applied

What information should be given to the patient?

In addition to being told about the expected effects of the treatment, the patient should be informed about possible side effects such as the painfulness of the application, bruises, etc. It is also important to warn the patient to report immediately any pain or discomfort experienced during the treatment (see also p. 18).

How often should flossing take place?

Flossing may be repeated several times in a single treatment session. After each application, the treated area should be allowed to recover completely. Simple movements, gentle, stroking massage and joint mobilization are a good idea during each break. Another flossing band application can be carried out after about 2–4 minutes, to achieve added benefit. If there is no further improvement, do not continue the treatment. The patient's tolerance is the defining factor for the frequency of the applications.

At what intervals should the treatments take place?

After-effects such as muscle soreness/stiffness and hematomas may occur after the first treatment session. The patient should be allowed sufficient recovery time. Depending on the after-effects, the treatment can continue the next day; otherwise, wait 2–3 days. If improvements are observed, it is best to start with the next treatment before any further deterioration sets in. If there is no improvement, or if the problem deteriorates, the treatment should be stopped.

Treating unpleasant after-effects

If skin irritation or transient pain develop after the flossing treatment, these may be treated using the simple "smoothing" technique. Grasp the previously flossed part of the body between thumb and index finger and push the muscle "away" with constant pressure (see Fig. 16). If necessary, repeat the technique 2–3 times.

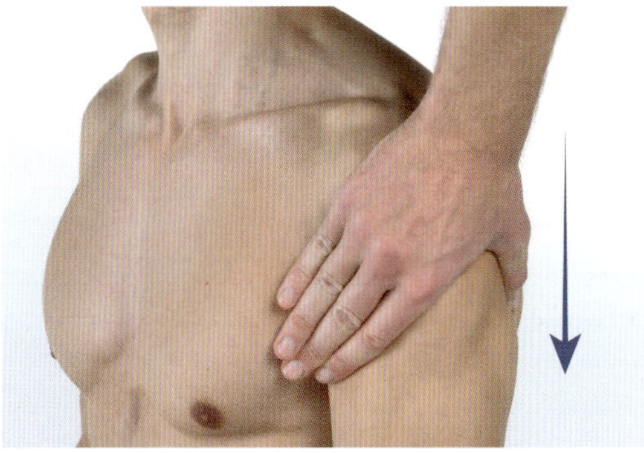

Fig. 16 Applying the smoothing technique on the upper arm.

General treatment tips

How many treatments are required?

This is a difficult question to answer. Basically, the longer the duration of the symptoms, the longer the therapy time that is required. There are many possibilities, from a single application to regular repetition. As described above, a follow-up intervention should always take place before any renewed deterioration sets in. Like so many treatment options in medicine, flossing is not a miracle cure and will not be effective against every problem.

Can it be combined with other forms of therapy?

The effect of flossing can be intensified with other exercises. Special exercises such as functional training, coordination exercises, stretches, or foam roller exercises for fascia release all show good results. If improved mobility is achieved, this should be maintained with regular exercises that utilize the full range of motion. In addition, the range of motion may be extended with the aid of joint manipulation therapy techniques.

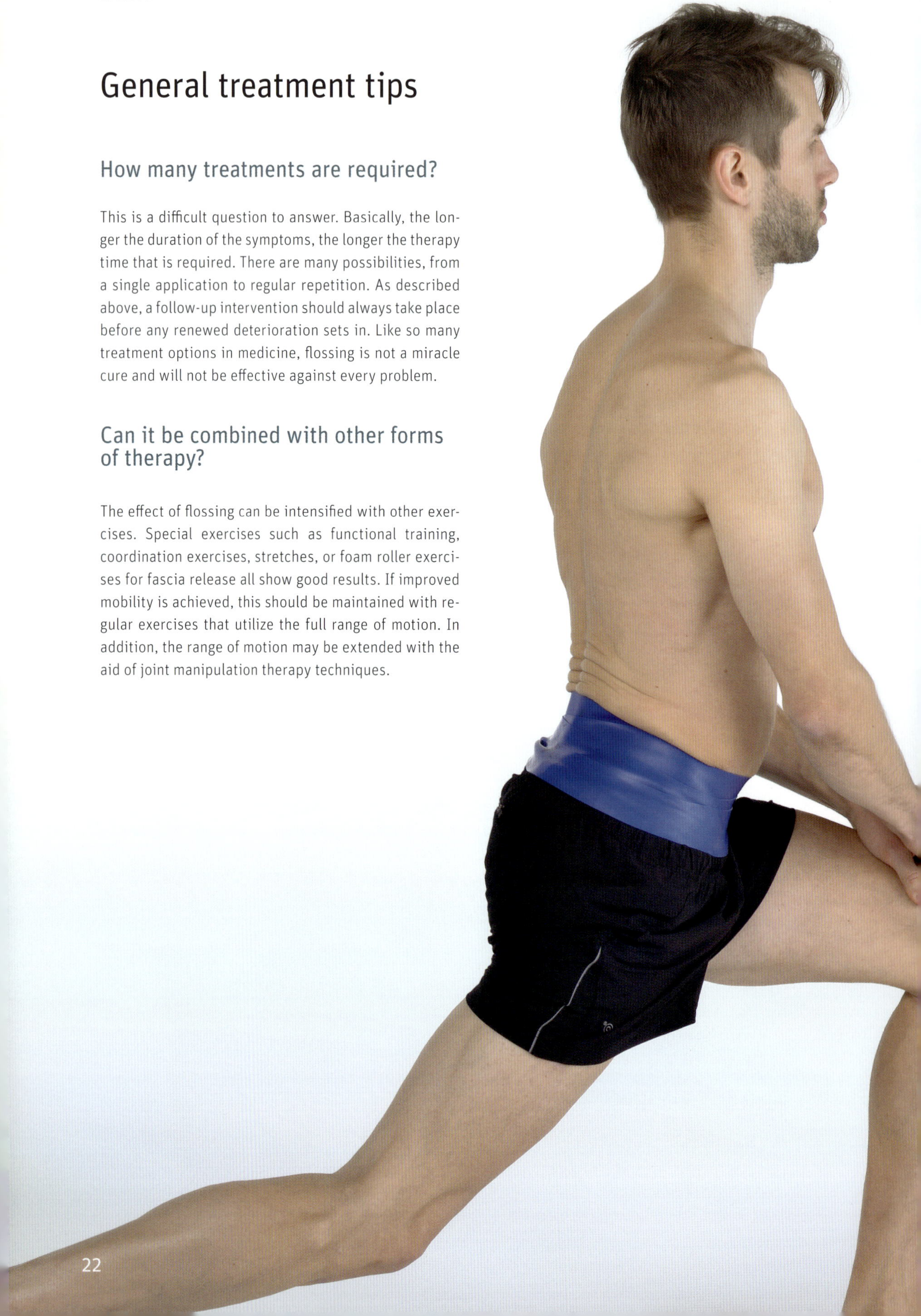

BFRT: Blood Flow Restriction Training

Flossing as strength training

In modified form, flossing band wraps can be used specifically for strength training. Variable compression wraps have been used in this way since the 1990's, the method becoming known as blood flow restriction training (BFRT, BFR training) and also as occlusion training.

BFRT means a form of training in which the blood flow to a muscle is reduced by the application of a compression bandage. As a result of this tourniquet, muscle exhaustion sets in more rapidly, followed by a marked increase in its strength and growth: the elastic bandages reduce the arterial blood supply, while the exercises are performed at low resistance. Binding off the muscle inhibits venous return, with only a slight restriction in arterial supply. This alters the muscle's biochemistry. In addition to the increase in lactate (lactic acid), there is reduction in pH, a low oxygen supply, swelling of the muscle cells and increased release of growth hormones. The muscle growth seen with low-resistance BFR training is approximates to that achieved by high-intensity training with heavy weights (70–80% of maximum strength). The positive effect of this training method has been particularly well-researched and demonstrated in recent years (Scott et al. 2015).

Since the exercises are performed at low resistance, this training method is particularly suitable for people who cannot or do not wish to exercise with heavy weights for health reasons. This may be the case following injuries or operations, or in arthritis and in elderly people (Abe et al. 2010, Ohta et al. 2003, Hylden et al. 2015). But even highly trained athletes can benefit from combining BFR training with standard training methods. In addition to its use in strength training, the increase in muscle strength and growth due to BFR training can also be achieved in low-intensity endurance sports such as walking and bicycling (Abe et al. 2006, 2010).

Flossing band wraps in strength training

Both areas of use, i.e. flossing to treat pain and flossing for strength training, involve movements performed with elastic bandages in place. However, there are some significant differences.

Note

Even though BFR training is regarded as safe, before using it you should talk to a physician or therapist about any contraindications (see p. 24).

- In strength training, the band is used to reduce blood supply and not to wrap the entire muscle. The recommendations from the meticulous study by Wilson (Wilson et al. 2013) should be applied here to ensure that flossing can be used without complications in both training and therapeutic practice.
- Only one width of the flossing band is applied above the relevant muscle. Thus, in contrast to flossing for the treatment of pain, compression is applied to a narrow area, not the entire muscle (see Fig. 18).
- The tension applied is uniform.
- The pressure should be perceived as firm, but should not cause any pain. For practical guidance, imagine a scale of 0 to 10 to allow you to assess the pressure produced by the band. 0 means no pressure at all and 10 stands for very powerful pressure with marked pain. The optimum score for the perceived pressure is around 7. This corresponds to pronounced compression without pain. Before you start regular training, you should familiarize yourself repeatedly with various pressure levels.

The BFR training procedure

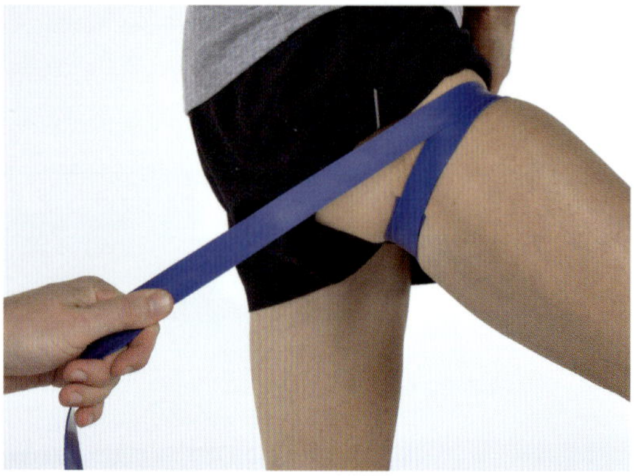

Fig. 18 Flossing band wrap for strength training applied to the upper thigh.

Contraindications and side effects

BFR training, whether self-applied or applied with assistance, requires a certain amount of instinctive feel and experience. The exercise protocol suggested here is based on guidelines from carefully conducted research studies and is regarded as very safe. The most common side effects are bruises, muscle stiffness/soreness and transient numbness. Contraindications include:

- Pregnancy
- A history of thrombosis
- Varicose veins
- Additional factors from the individual's medical history (see p. 17)

How strong should the resistance be?

Low-resistance exercises are performed while the muscle is tied off. These should be equivalent to 20% (ranging between 15–30%) of maximum resistance, i.e. the person exercising should be capable of repeating the exercise in question 50–70 times when the muscle is not tied off. Depending on the exercise, the resistance may be produced with the aid of light free weights, training machines set at low resistance or with one's own body (see Fig. 19 and 20). According to study results, exercises that load several joints are preferable. This also leads to increased strength.of the trunk muscles (Yasuda et al. 2010).

How many sets are required?

Four to five sets of low-resistance exercises are performed, but with only 15–30 repetitions. There should be 30 repetitions in the first set and only 15 each in sets 2–4. Breaks of 30 seconds to one minute should be taken between the sets. The wrap is kept in place throughout the exercise period and removed only after the last set is completed. At the start of training, exhaustion may already set in before the number of suggested repetitions has been reached.

How often should training take place?

2–3 training units per week are sufficient for rehabilitation training or if there are existing health problems. Highly athletic individuals can include 2–4 units of BFR training into their program in addition to their usual training workload.

BFR TRAINING BASICS – AN OVERWIEW

- A single turn of the band close to the groin or axilla, wound at uniform tension
- Clearly perceptible compression without pain (perceived tourniquet pressure of 7 on a scale of 0 to 10)
- Perform 4–5 sets of low-resistance exercises
- First set with 30 repetitions, subsequent sets with 15 repetitions each or until fatigue sets in (30–15–15–15–15)
- Breaks of 30 seconds to one minute between sets
- The bandage is not removed until after the last set
- If pain develops, the training should be stopped

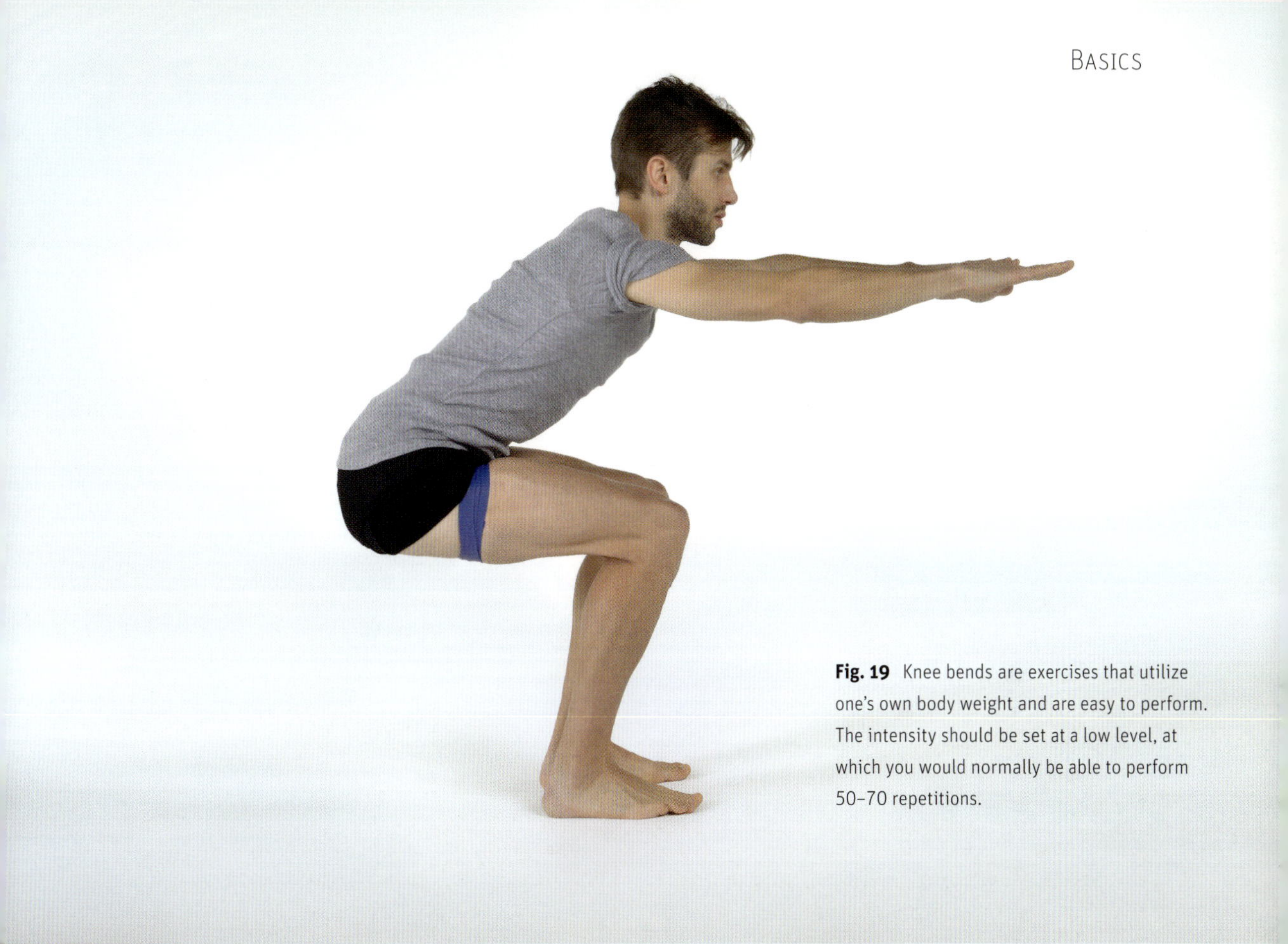

Fig. 19 Knee bends are exercises that utilize one's own body weight and are easy to perform. The intensity should be set at a low level, at which you would normally be able to perform 50–70 repetitions.

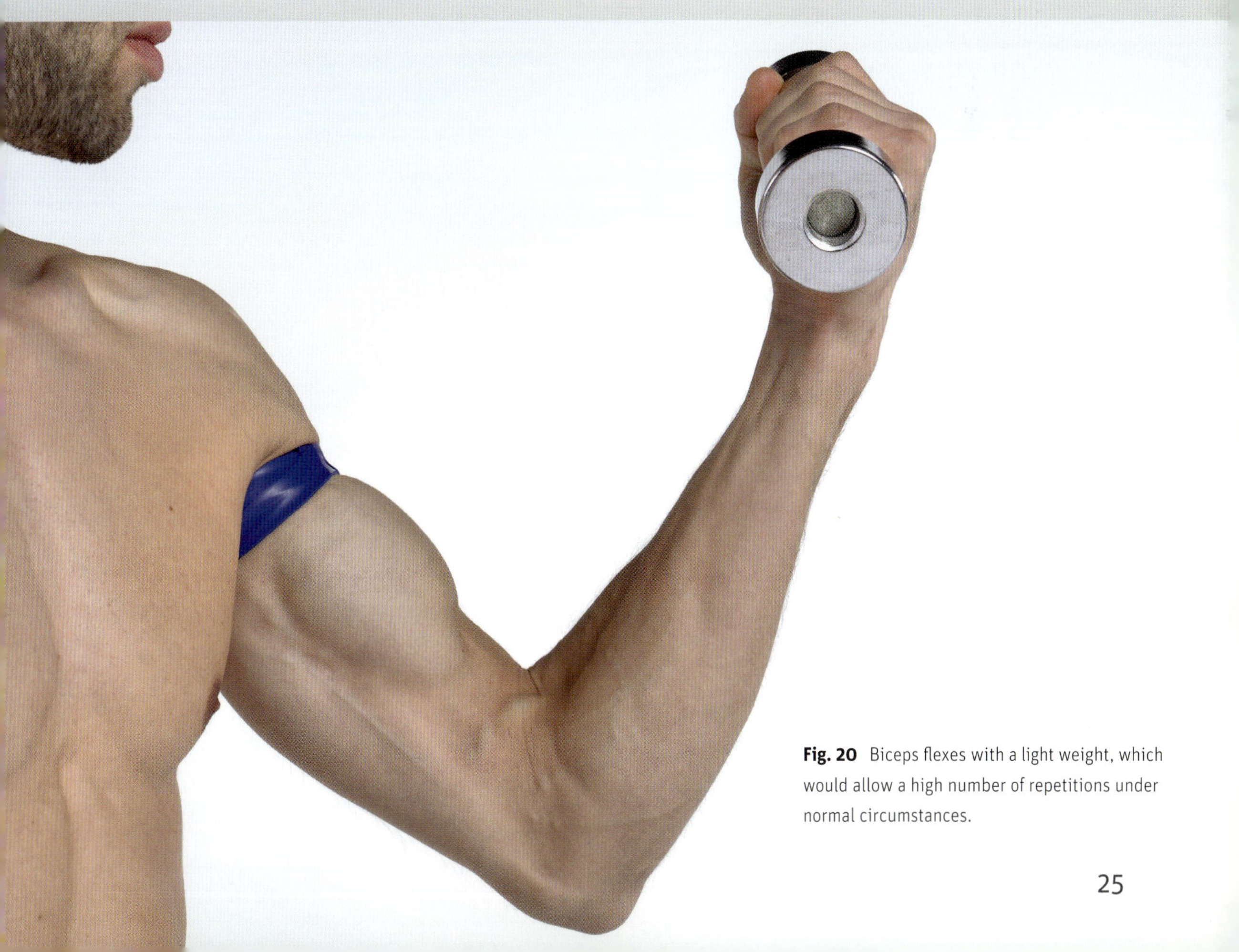

Fig. 20 Biceps flexes with a light weight, which would allow a high number of repetitions under normal circumstances.

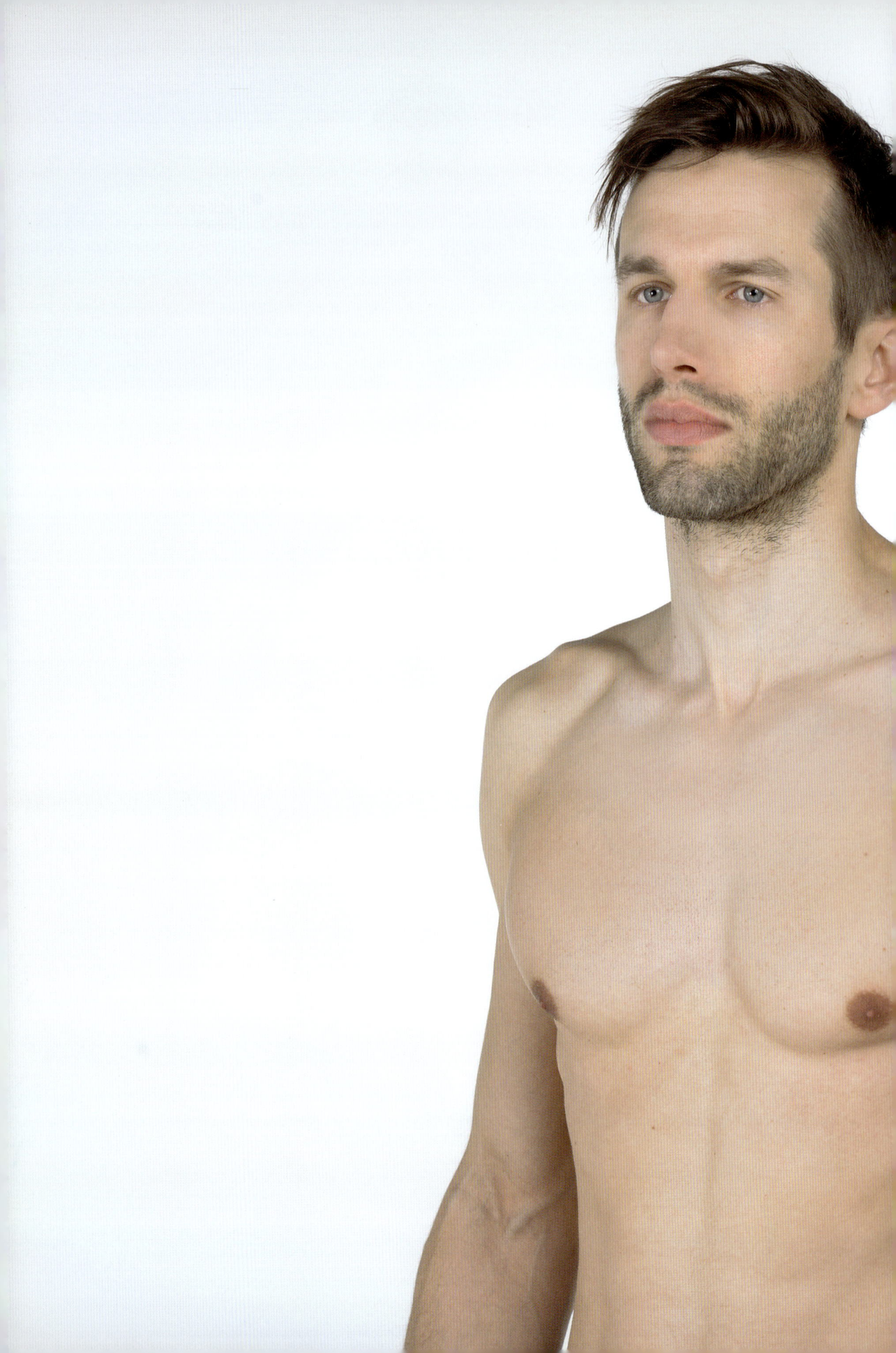

FLOSSING – THE PRACTICE

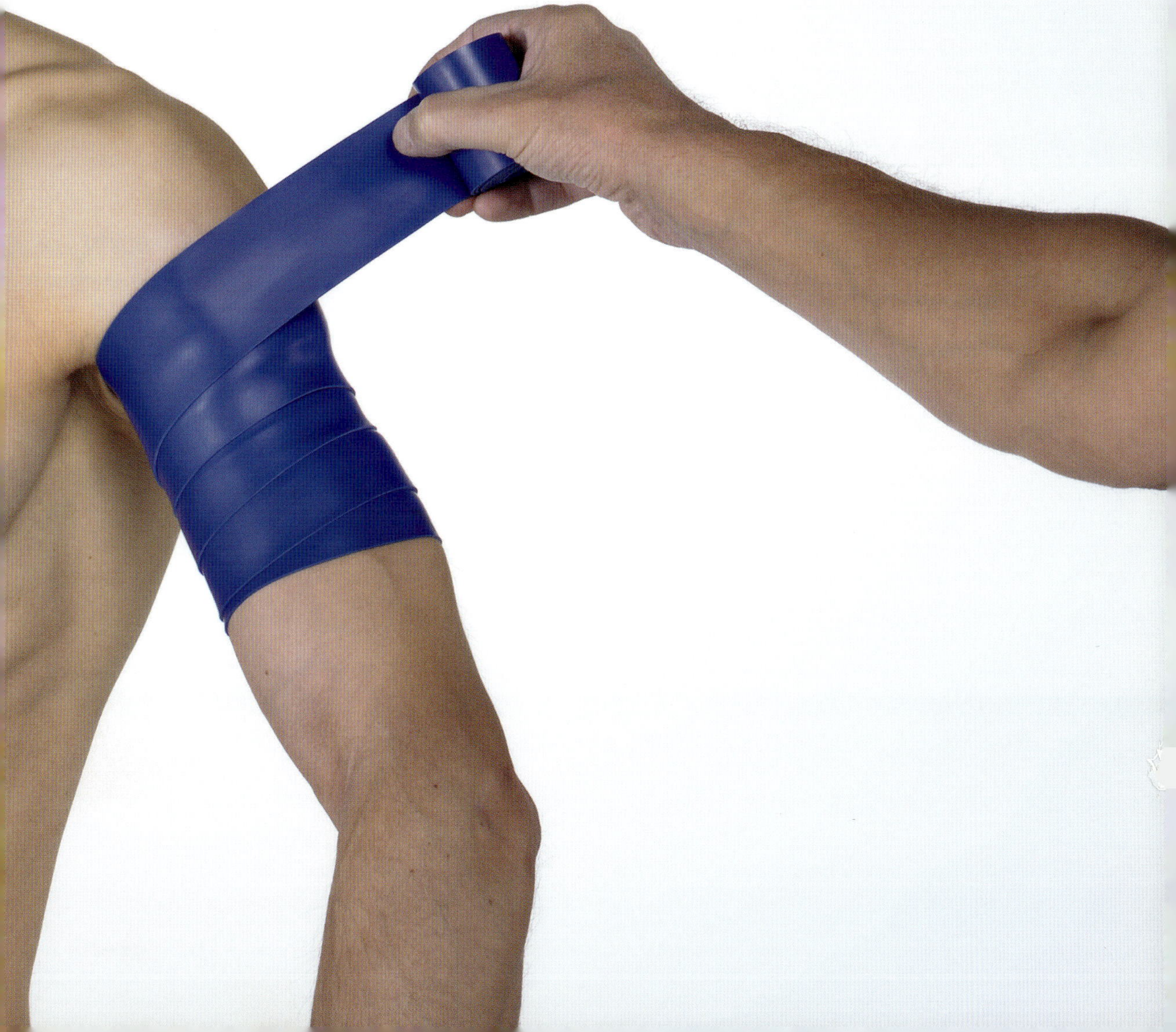

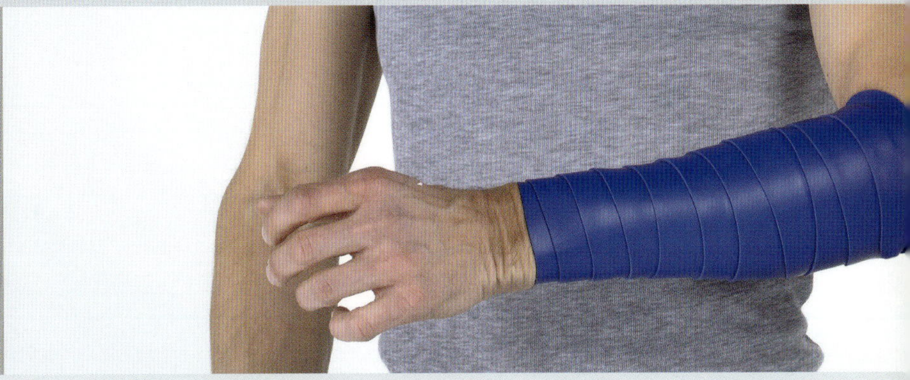

CHAPTER 1:

FLOSSING BAND WRAPS FOR UPPER EXTREMITY PAIN

Acromioclavicular joint

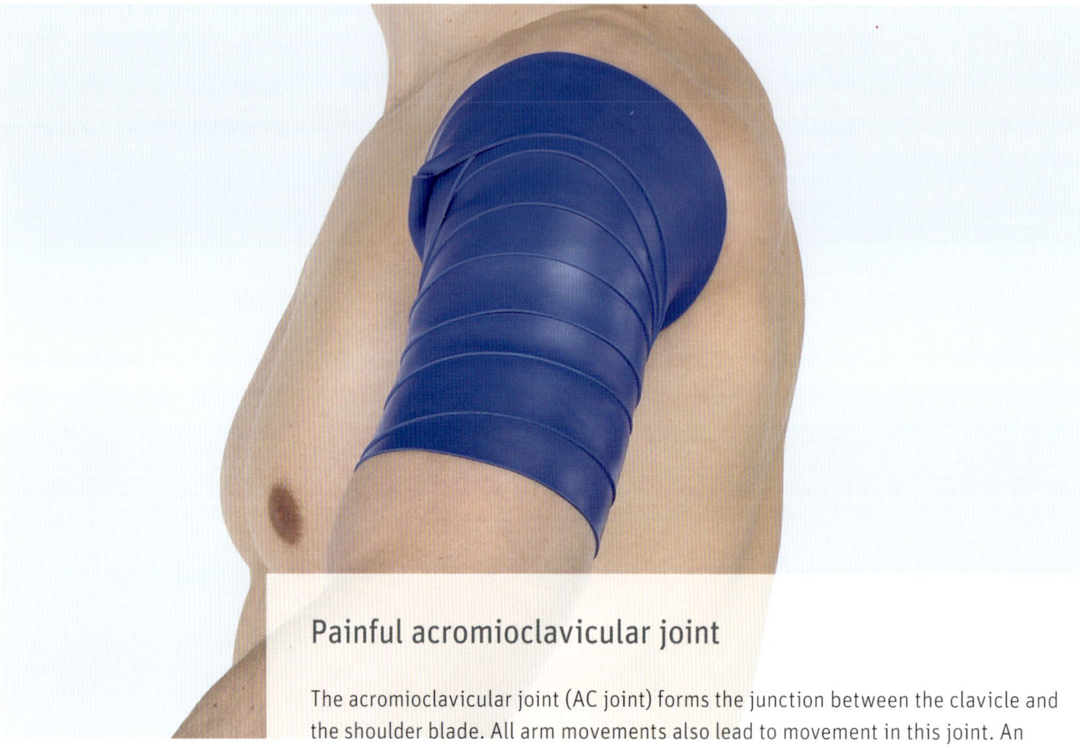

Painful acromioclavicular joint

The acromioclavicular joint (AC joint) forms the junction between the clavicle and the shoulder blade. All arm movements also lead to movement in this joint. An injury to the AC joint is therefore associated with pain whenever any extensive arm movements are performed. In most cases, injuries to this joint involve tearing of the surrounding ligaments, usually occurring following a fall directly onto the shoulder and also as a result of severe strain to the pectoral girdle (e.g. handstand in gymnasts).

The flossing band wrap ⇢ Here's how it works

1 The patient's arm is abducted and held either laterally or extended forwards, with the hand supported on the therapy couch. Wind the first turn with 50% tension to anchor the band around the upper part of the upper arm.

2 Now continue winding the flossing band in ascending circular turns. The band should overlap 50% at each turn. A tension of 60–80% should be applied particularly to the outer side of the upper arm and to the AC joint.

3 Using the same technique, wind the band as far up over the shoulder as possible and secure it into place.

Painful movement

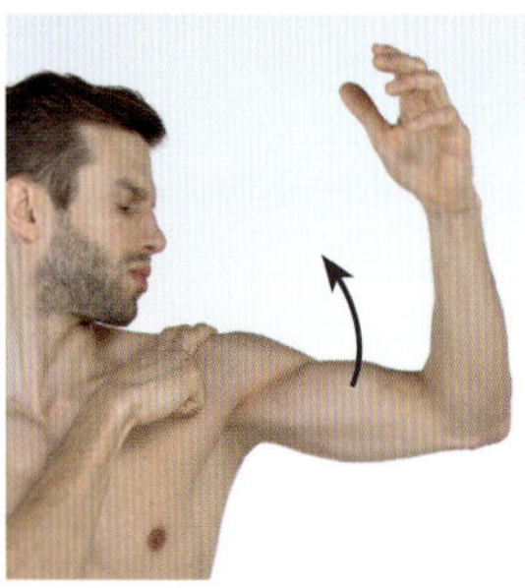

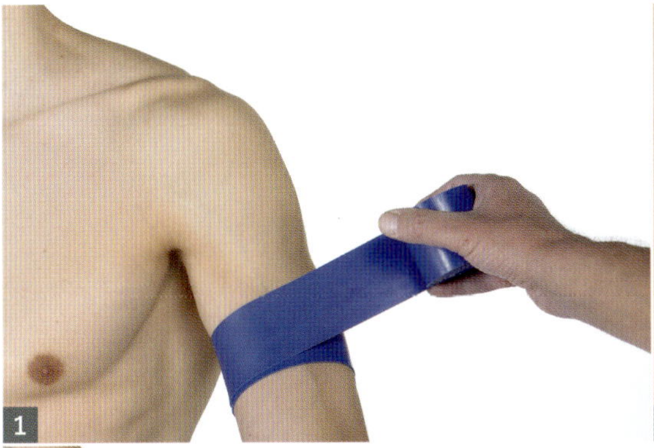

1

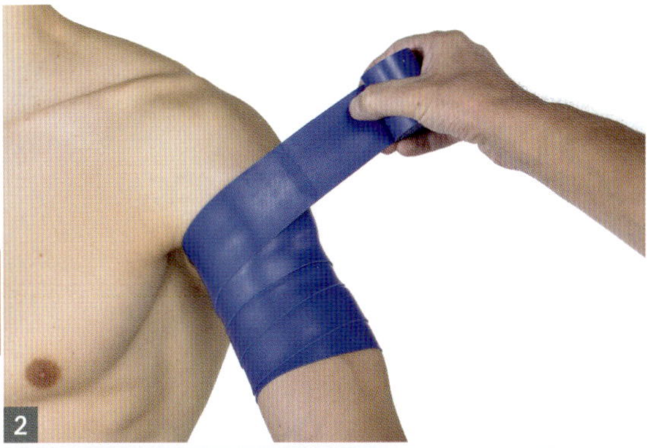

2

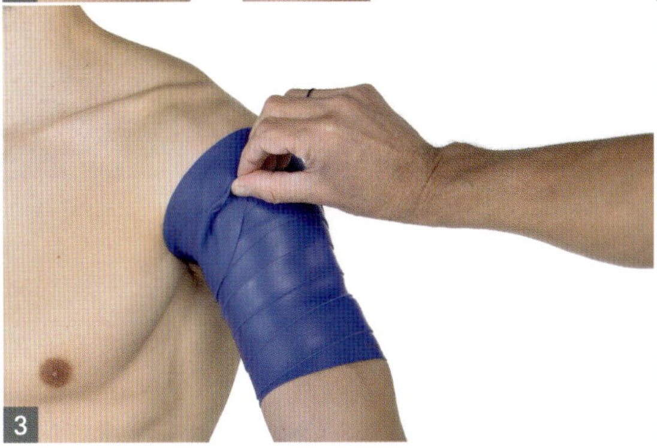

3

Material: Flossing band
Length: 2.06 m
Width: 5 cm
Tension: outside/top 60–80%, inside 50%

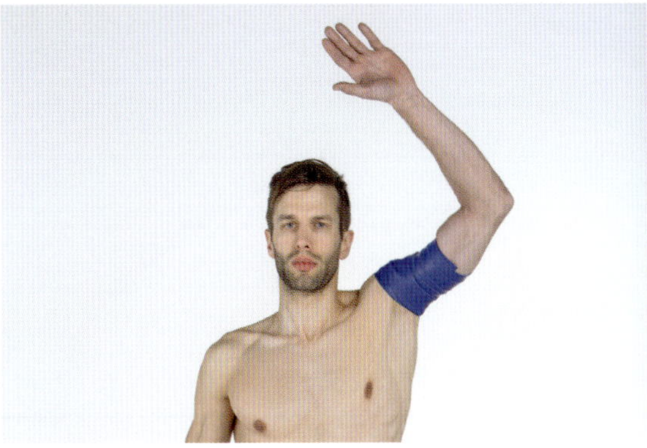

Active Exercise

Perform movements with the pectoral girdle and arm, making them as extensive as possible. Make sure that you move in all directions, particularly external rotation. A shoulder pulley device or a Thera-Band® may also be used for this purpose.

A Word of Advice > The first flossing treatment of the upper arm should be applied with slightly reduced band tension (max. 60%), since transient pain and/or numbness may sometimes be experienced after the treatment. Direct compressive and tensile strains on the joint should be avoided (sleeping on the shoulder, heavy lifting and carrying).

Shoulder, shoulder stiffness, impingement syndrome

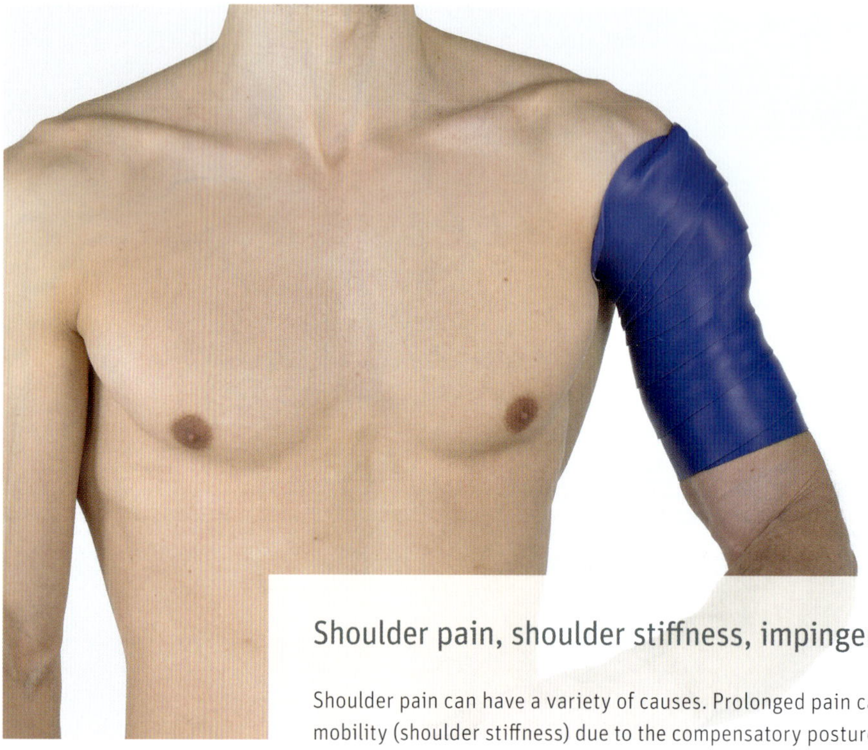

Shoulder pain, shoulder stiffness, impingement syndrome

Shoulder pain can have a variety of causes. Prolonged pain can lead to restricted mobility (shoulder stiffness) due to the compensatory posture adopted by the sufferer. Muscular imbalance or overhead work may lead to compression of the supraspinatus tendon with resultant impingement syndrome.

The flossing band wrap ⇢ Here's how it works

1 The patient's arm is abducted and held either laterally or extended forwards, with the hand supported on the therapy couch. Wind the first turn with 50% tension to anchor the band around the upper part of the upper arm.

2 Now wind the flossing band in ascending circular turns. The band should overlap 50% at each turn. A tension of 60–80% should be applied to the shoulder joint and acromion, with a tension of 50% on the posterior side of the shoulder.

3 Using the same technique, wind the band as far up as possible and secure it into place.

Painful movement

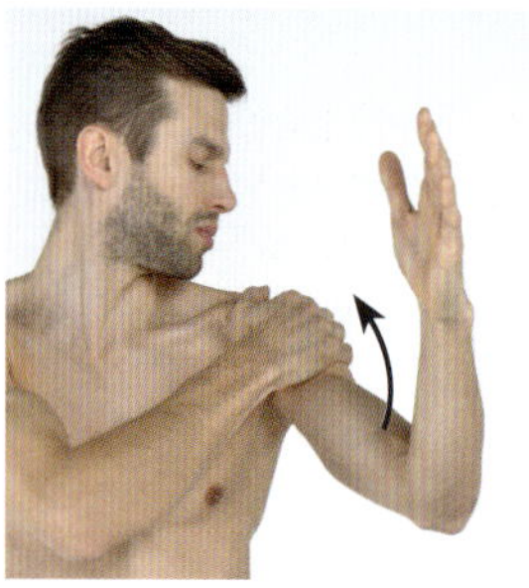

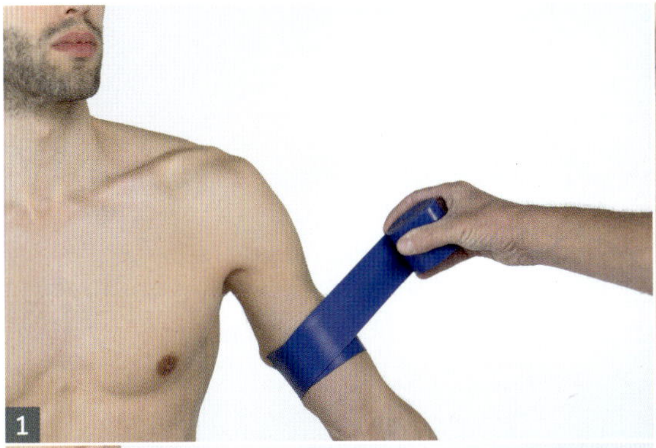

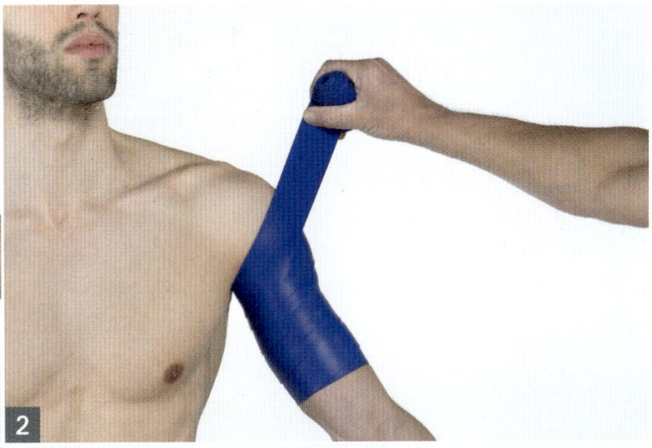

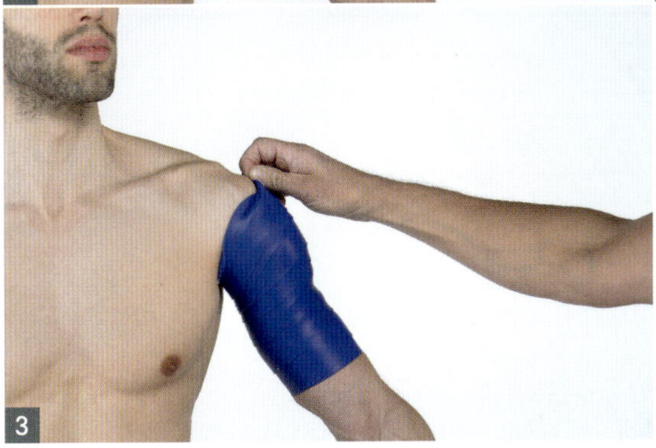

Material: Flossing band
Length: 2.06 m
Width: 5 cm
Tension: front 60–80%, back 50%

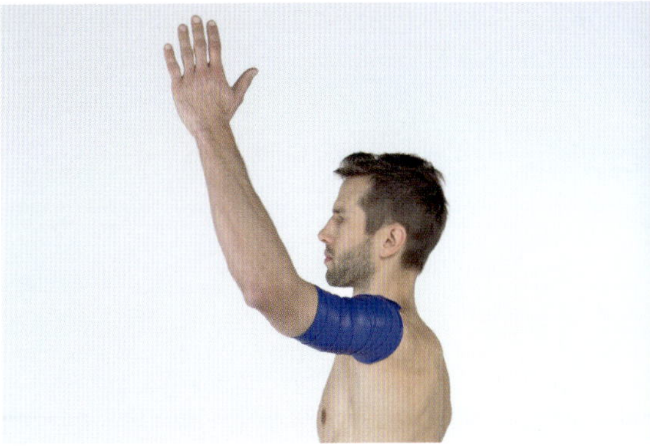

Active Exercise

Perform movements with the arm, making them as extensive as possible. Make sure that you move in all directions, particularly external rotation. A shoulder pulley device or a Thera-Band® may also be used for this purpose. You can do push-ups on the therapy couch to intensify the exercise.

A Word of Advice > The first flossing treatment of the upper arm should be applied with slightly reduced band tension (max. 60%), since transient pain and/or numbness may sometimes be experienced after the treatment. If there is any tendon pain in the shoulder region, strength sports and intensive lifting and carrying should be avoided.

Biceps muscle and long biceps tendon

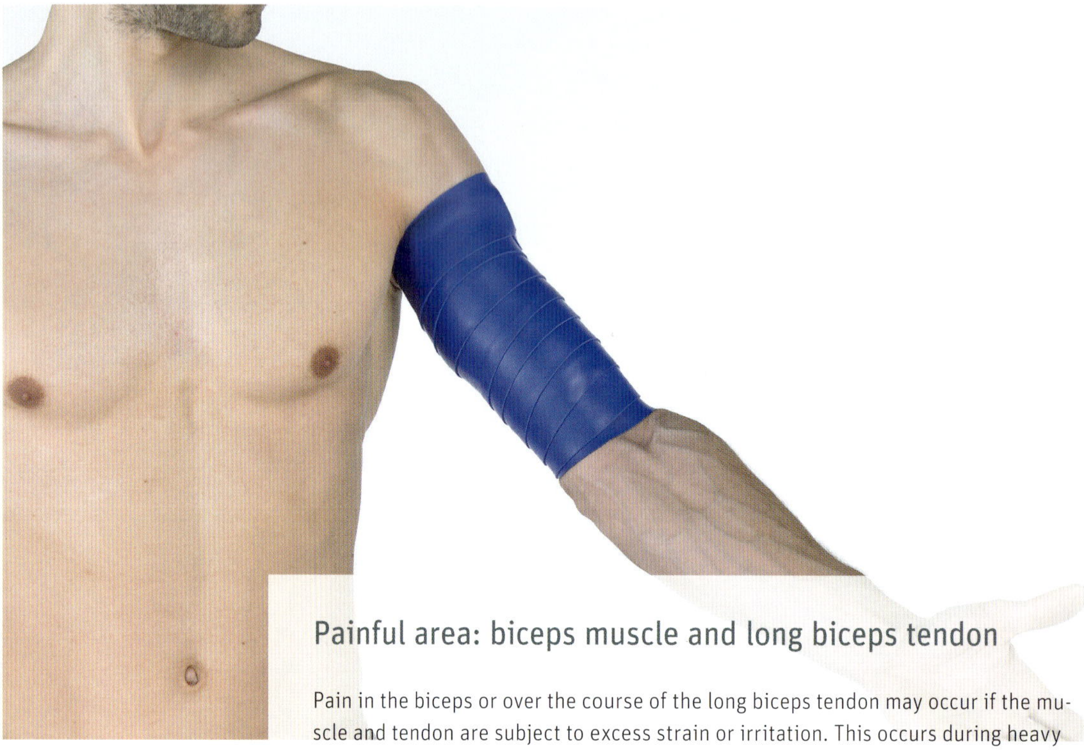

Painful area: biceps muscle and long biceps tendon

Pain in the biceps or over the course of the long biceps tendon may occur if the muscle and tendon are subject to excess strain or irritation. This occurs during heavy lifting and carrying activities and also in sports (strength training). The tendon is often very painful near the shoulder joint.

The flossing band wrap ⇢ Here's how it works

1 The patient's elbow joint is extended, with the hand supported on the therapy couch. Wind the first turn with 50% tension to anchor the band around the lower part of the upper arm.

2 Now wind the flossing band in ascending circular turns. The band should overlap 50% at each turn. A tension of 60–80% should be applied to the biceps muscle and the long biceps tendon, with a tension of 50% on the posterior side of the upper arm.

3 Using the same technique, wind the band up to the shoulder and secure it into place close to the shoulder joint.

Painful movement

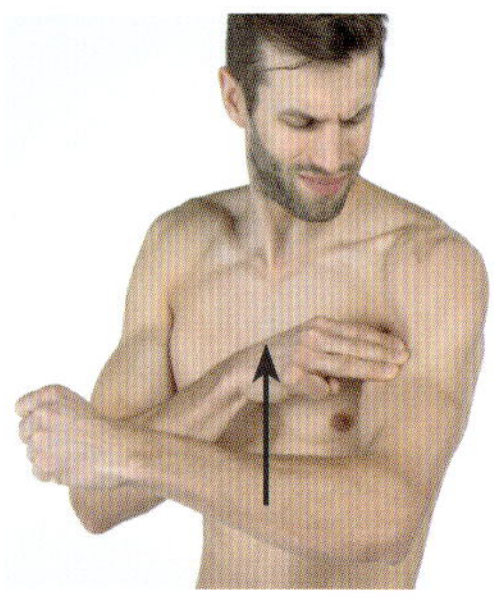

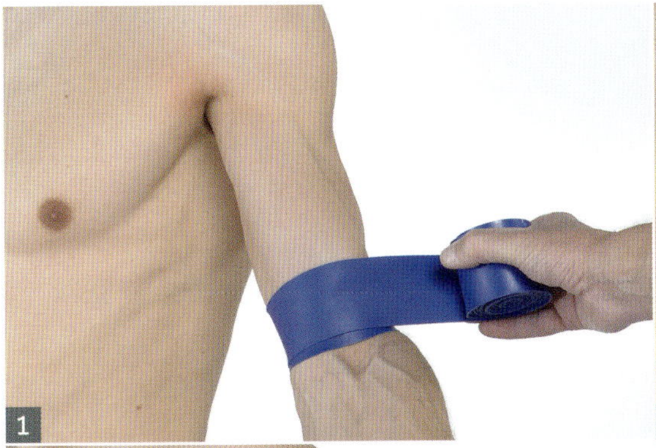

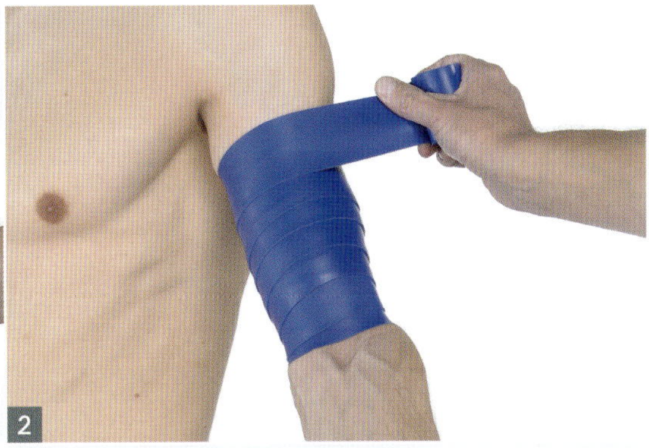

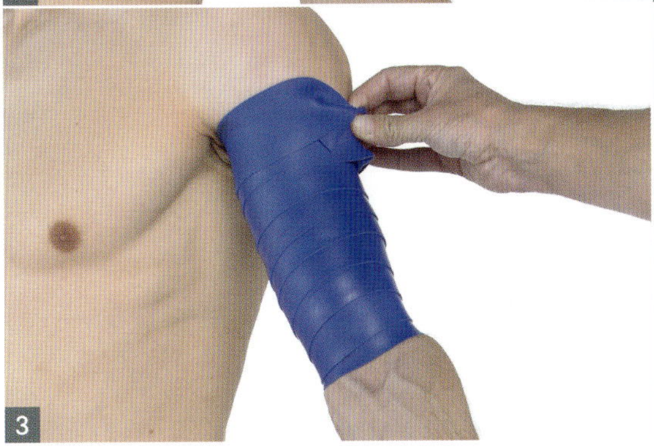

Material: Flossing band
Length: 2.06 m
Width: 5 cm
Tension: front 60–80%, back 50%

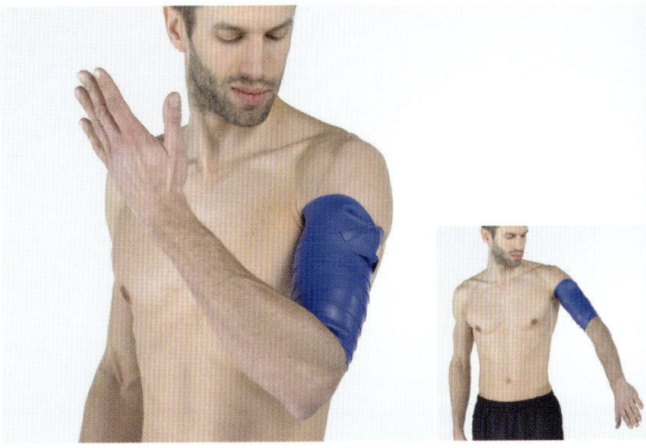

Active Exercise

Extend and flex the elbow maximally and rotate the forearm inwards and outwards. Follow this with extensive forward and backward movements of the arm. To intensify the exercise, lift an object up several times or do push-ups.

A Word of Advice > The first flossing treatment of the upper arm should be applied with slightly reduced band tension (max. 60%), since transient pain and/or numbness may sometimes be experienced after the treatment. If there is any tendon pain in the shoulder region, strength sports and intensive lifting and carrying should be avoided.

Upper arm fascia

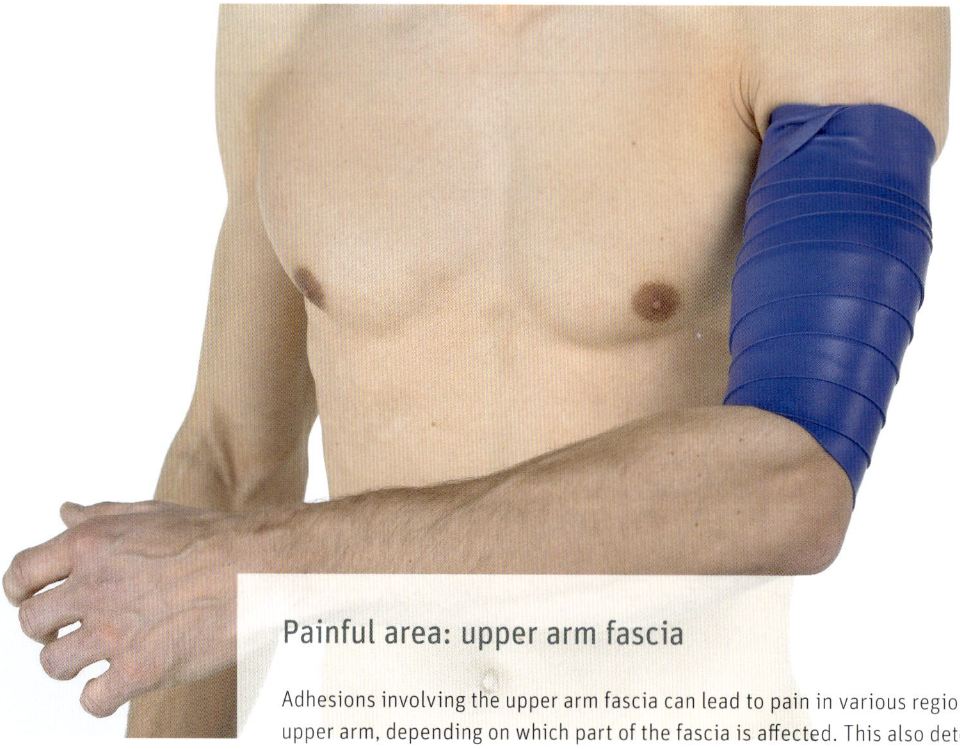

Painful area: upper arm fascia

Adhesions involving the upper arm fascia can lead to pain in various regions of the upper arm, depending on which part of the fascia is affected. This also determines the technique used to apply the flossing band wrap.

The flossing band wrap ⇢ Here's how it works

1 The patient's elbow joint is extended, with the hand supported on the therapy couch. Wind the first turn with 50% tension to anchor the band around the lower part of the upper arm.

2 Now wind the flossing band in ascending circular turns. The band should overlap 50% at each turn. A tension of 60–80% should be applied in the regions of the adhesions and painful fascia, with a tension of 50% on the other side of the upper arm.

3 Using the same technique, wind the band up to the shoulder and secure it into place close to the shoulder joint.

Where it hurts on movement

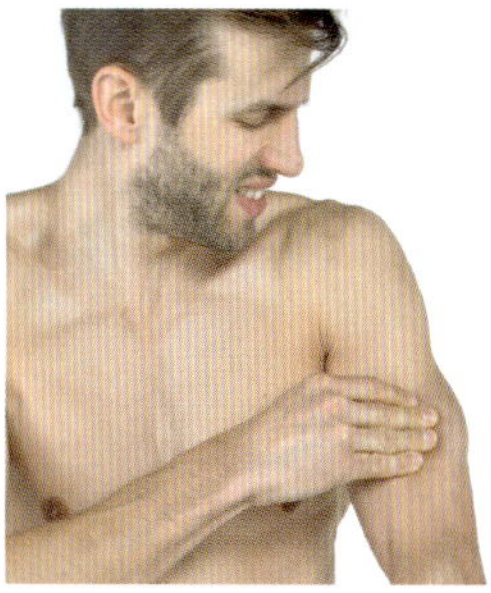

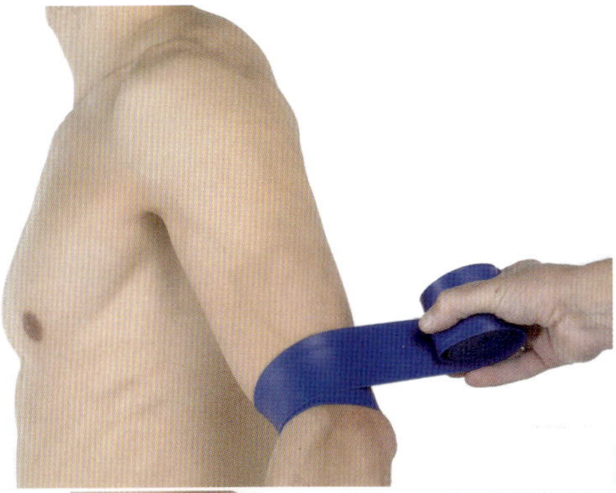

1

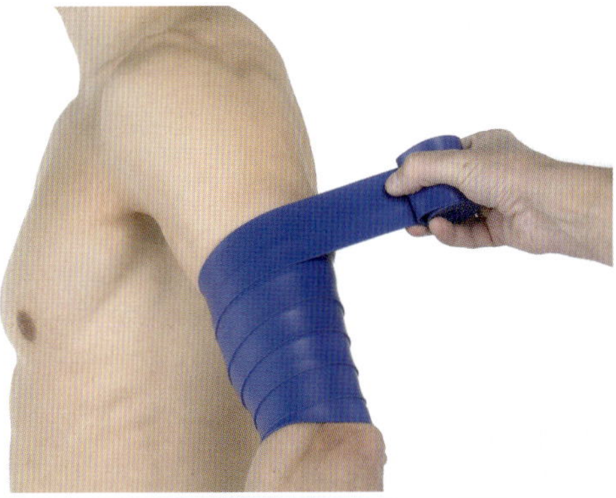

2

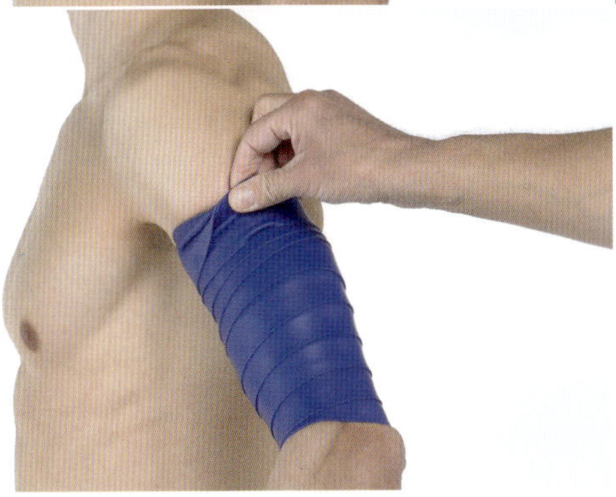

3

Material: Flossing band
Length: 2.06 m
Width: 5 cm
Tension: painful region 60–80%, other side 50%

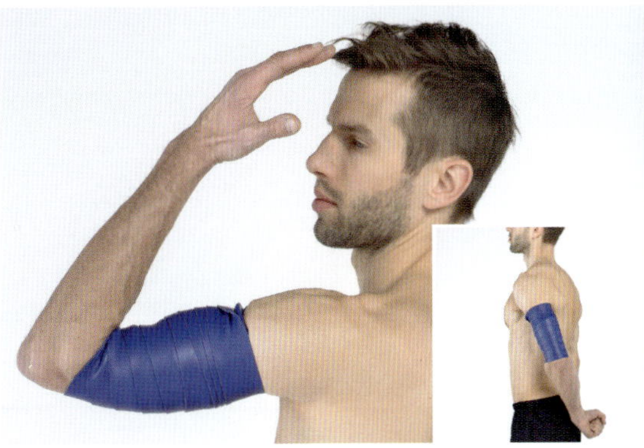

Active Exercise

Extend and flex the elbow maximally and rotate the forearm inwards and outwards. Follow this with extensive forward and backward movements of the arm.

A Word of Advice > Smooth, steady movements in the shoulder and elbow joints, performed using little strength, can help loosen the adhesions (e.g. swimming).

Elbow joint

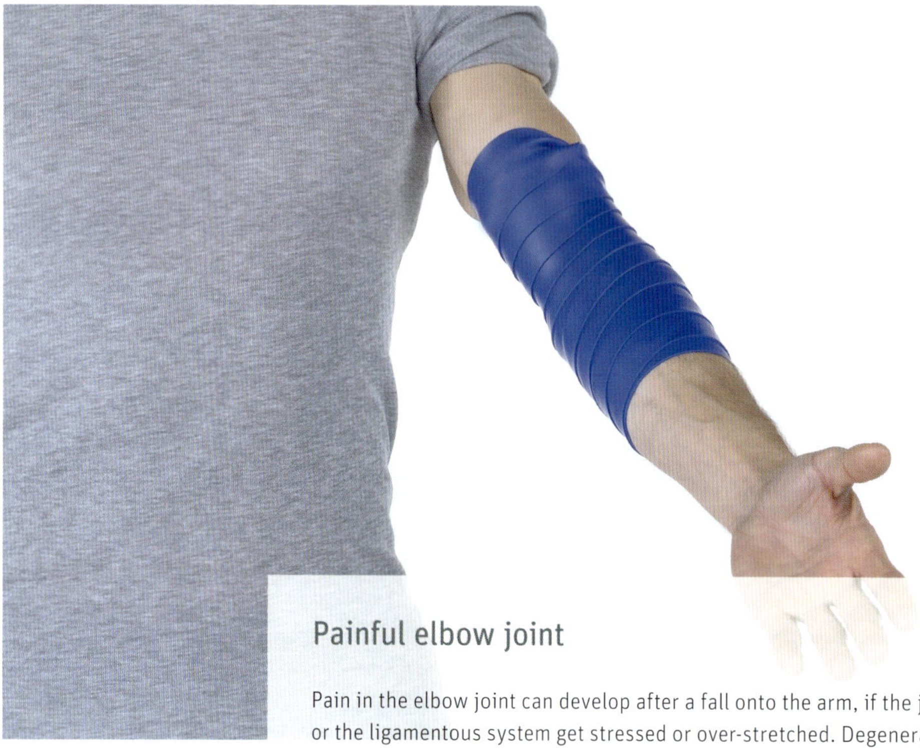

Painful elbow joint

Pain in the elbow joint can develop after a fall onto the arm, if the joint capsule or the ligamentous system get stressed or over-stretched. Degenerative arthritic changes or irritation of the ligaments can also lead to pain.

The flossing band wrap ⇢ Here's how it works

1 The patient's elbow joint is extended. Wind the first turn with 50% tension to anchor the band around the upper part of the forearm.

2 Now wind the flossing band in ascending circular turns. The band should overlap 50% at each turn. A tension of 60–80% should be applied at the elbow flexure or over the painful ligaments (depending on the main location of the pain), with a tension of 50% on the other side of the arm.

3 Using the same technique, wind the band up to the middle of the upper arm and secure it into place there.

Where it hurts on movement

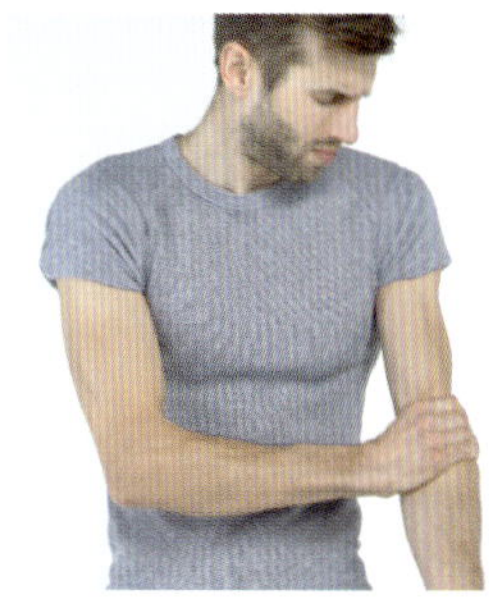

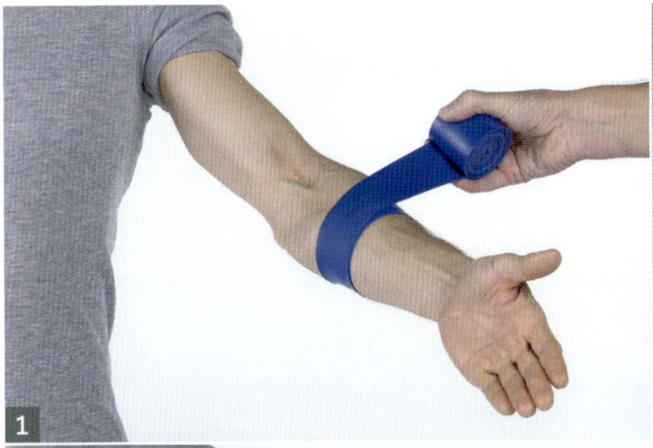

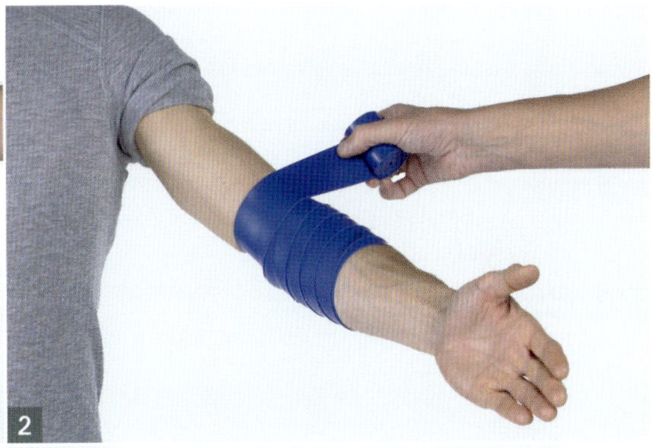

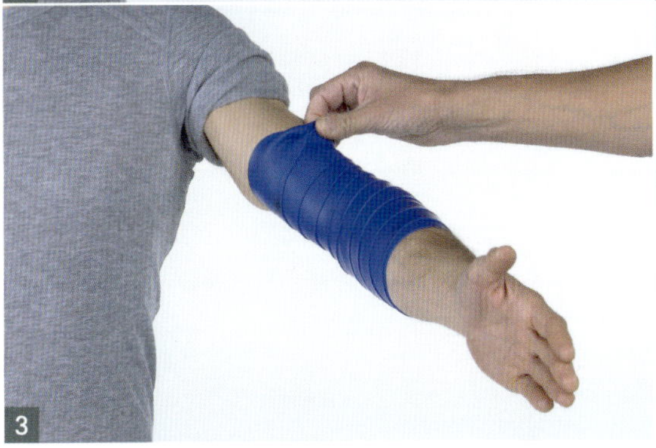

Material: Flossing band
Length: 2.06 m
Width: 5 cm
Tension: Painful site 60–80%, other side 50%

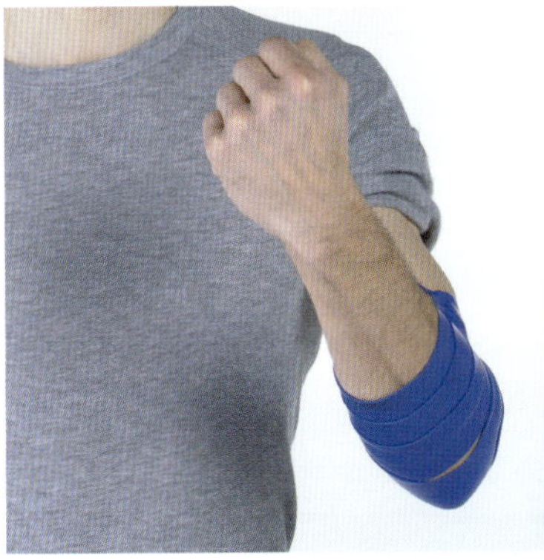

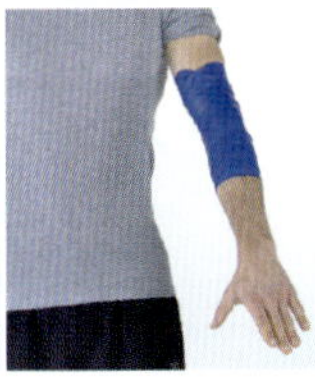

Active Exercise

Extend and flex the elbow maximally and rotate the forearm inwards and outwards. This can be followed by half push-ups on the therapy couch, over the desk, or against the wall.

A Word of Advice > If there is pain in the collateral ligaments of the elbow joint, the tension applied over the painful region should be 60–80%. For this purpose, the flossing band may also be wrapped over the painful region in "crisscross" turns.

Tennis elbow

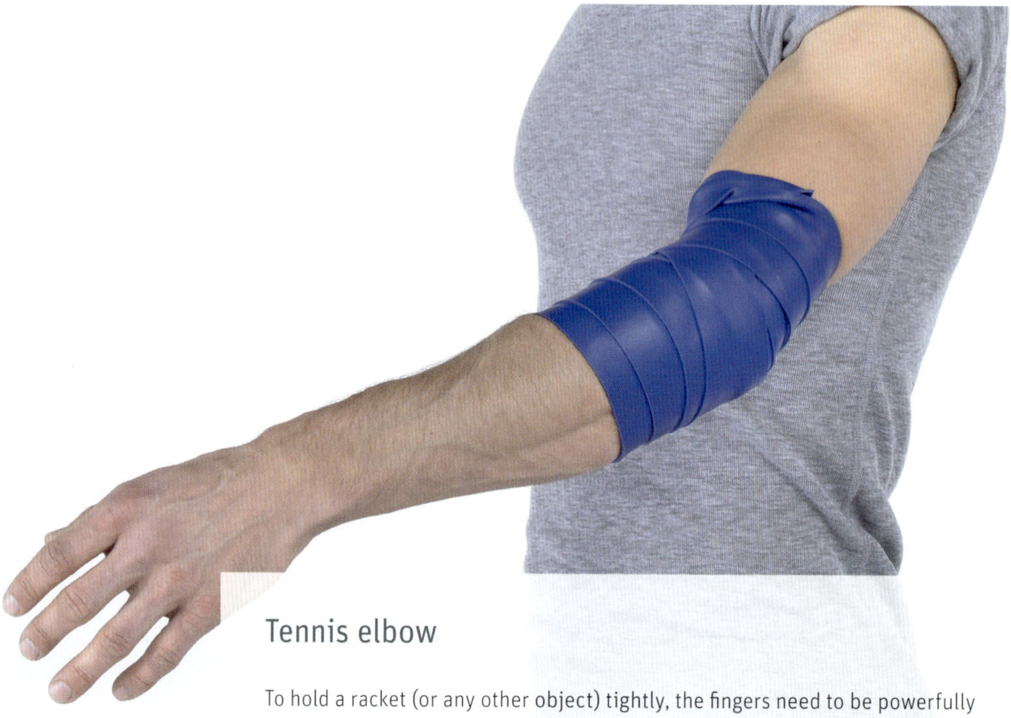

Tennis elbow

To hold a racket (or any other object) tightly, the fingers need to be powerfully flexed and the wrist joint pulled up slightly. Tennis elbow involves strain and irritation of the muscles that pull up the wrist joint. These muscles are located on the outer side of forearm, while the tendon from which they originate is attached laterally at the elbow. In general, the most severe pain is also experienced in this region.

The flossing band wrap ⇢ Here's how it works

1 The patient's elbow joint is extended. Wind the first turn with 50% tension to anchor the band around the upper part of the forearm.

2 Now wind the flossing band in ascending circular turns. The band should overlap 50% at each turn. A tension of 60–80% should be applied over the outer elbow, with a tension of 50% over the inner elbow.

3 Using the same technique, wind the band up to the middle of the upper arm; if required, the band can also be crossed over again above the painful region (step 2, small image). Secure it into place on the upper arm.

Where it hurts on movement

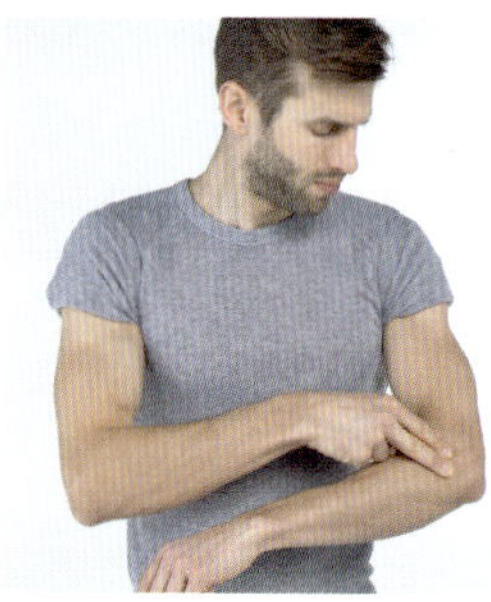

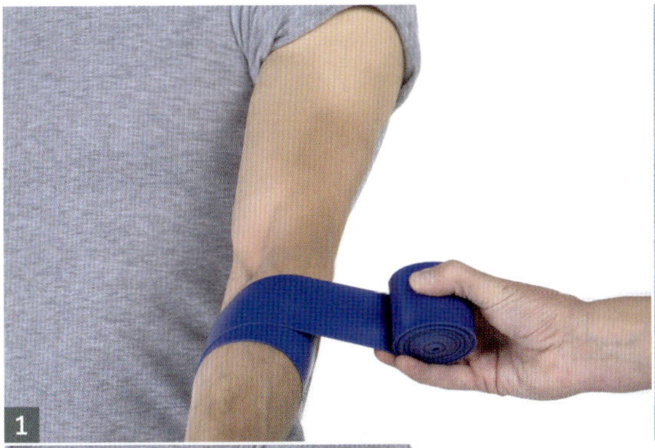

1

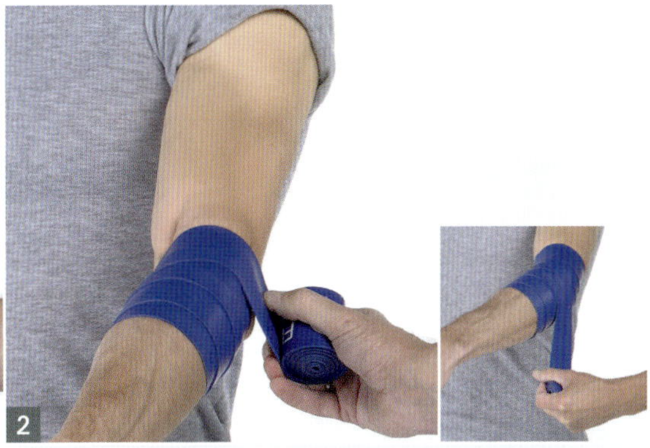

2

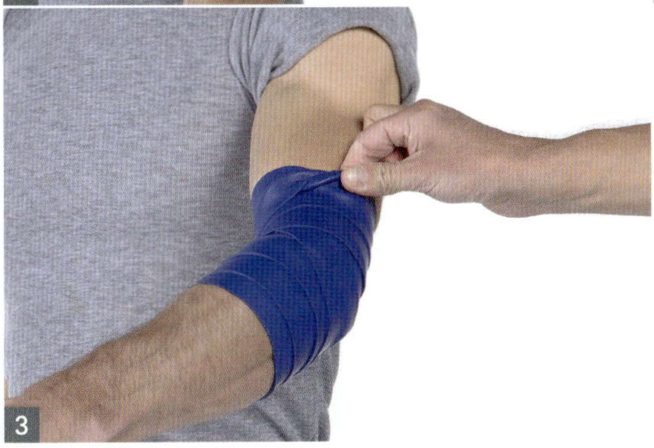

3

Material: Flossing band
Length: 2.06 m
Width: 5 cm
Tension: Outside 60–80%, inside 50%

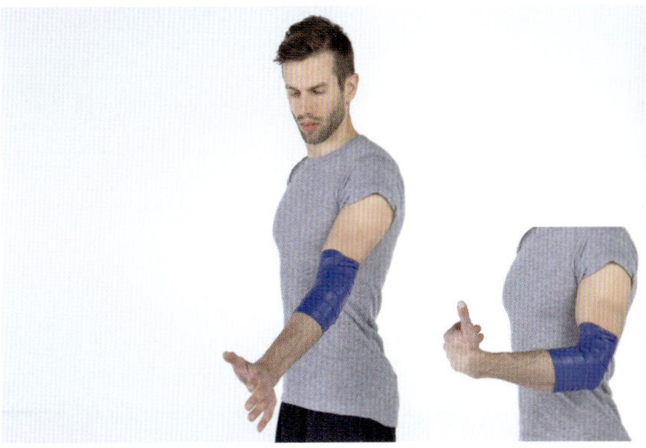

Active Exercise

Make a loose fist and stretch the finger maximally. After this, move the wrist maximally into flexion and loosely into extension. Then flex and extend the elbow, and rotate the forearm both inwards and outwards.

A Word of Advice > To release and relax the muscles, you should move the wrist joint extensively, but without much force in the painful area. The application of heat (warm bath, sauna, etc.) increases blood flow and aids regeneration.

Golfer's elbow

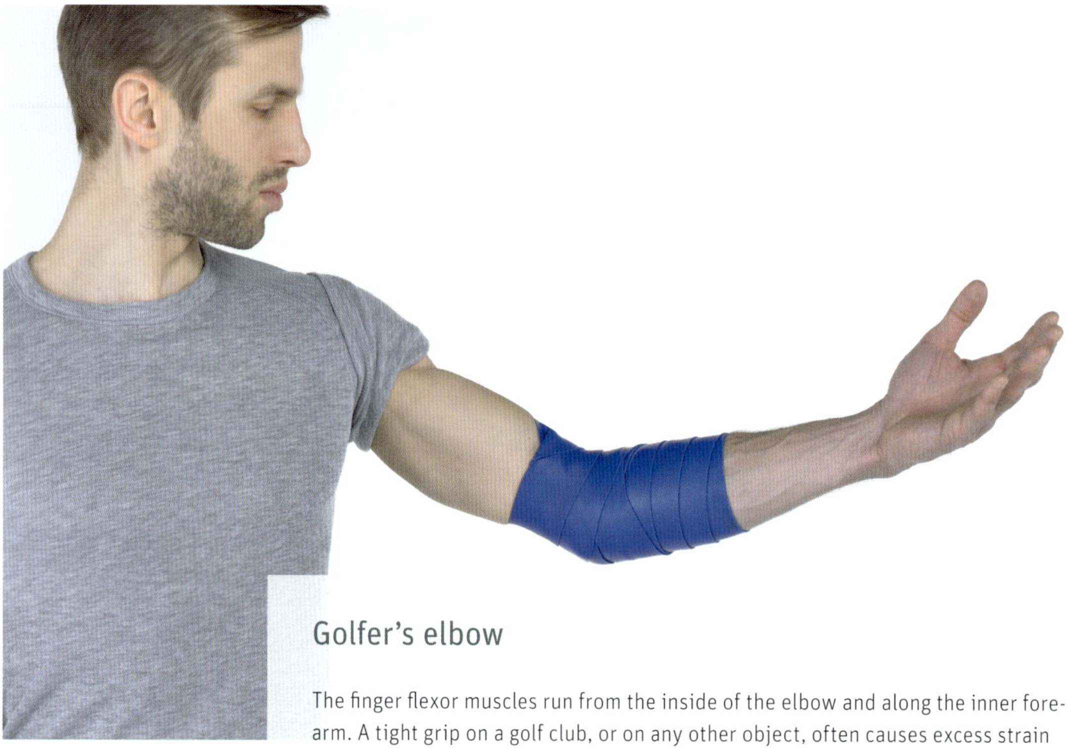

Golfer's elbow

The finger flexor muscles run from the inside of the elbow and along the inner forearm. A tight grip on a golf club, or on any other object, often causes excess strain on these muscles. Golfer's elbow involves strain and irritation of the muscles that flex the fingers and wrist joint. The most severe pain generally occurs in the inner elbow region.

The flossing band wrap ⇢ Here's how it works

1 The patient's elbow joint is extended. Wind the first turn with 50% tension to anchor the band around the upper part of the forearm.

2 Now wind the flossing band in ascending circular turns. The band should overlap 50% at each turn. A tension of 60–80% should be applied over the inner elbow, with a tension of 50% over the outer elbow.

3 Using the same technique, wind the band up to the middle of the upper arm; if required, the band can also be crossed over again above the painful region (step 2, small image). Fix the band into place on the upper arm.

Where it hurts on movement

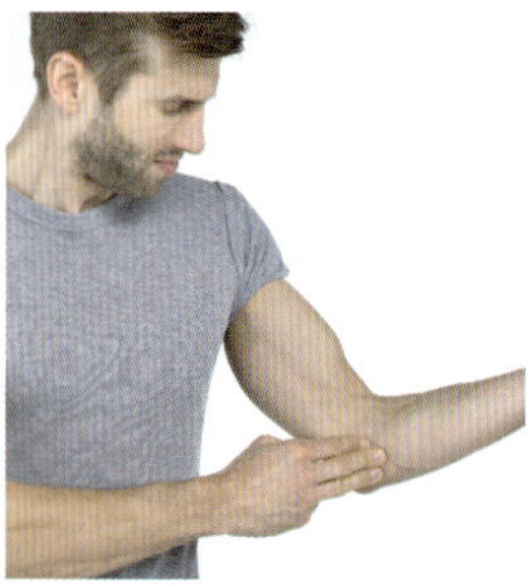

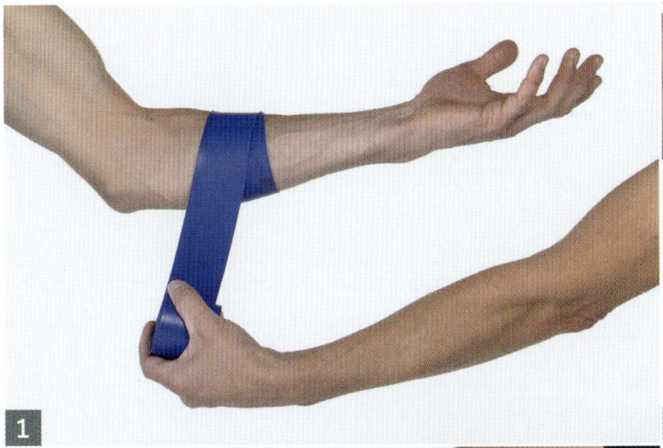

1

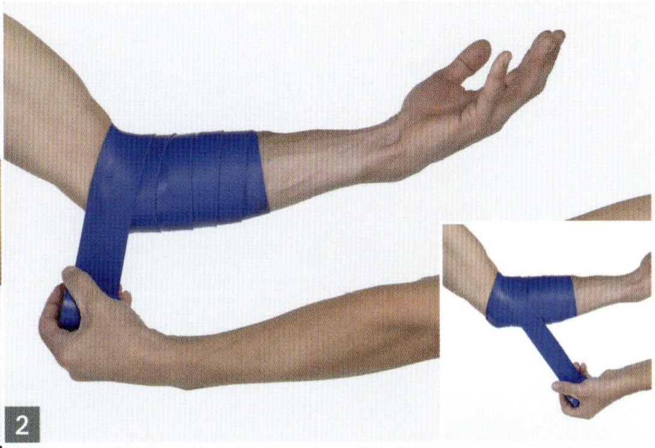

2

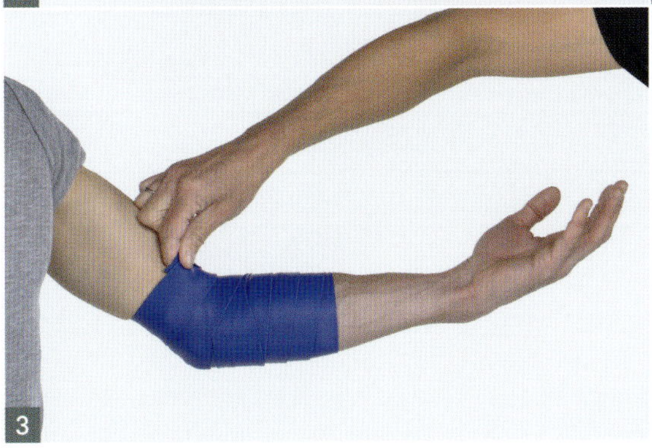

3

Material: Flossing band
Length: 2.06 m
Width: 5 cm
Tension: Inside 60–80%, outside 50%

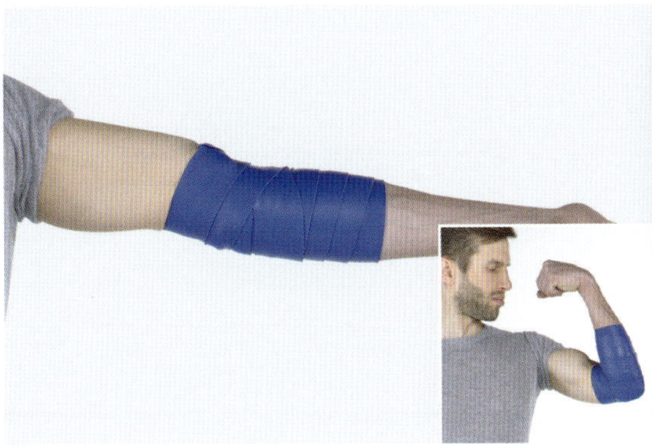

Active Exercise

Make a loose fist and stretch the finger maximally. After this, move the wrist loosely into flexion and maximally into extension. Then flex and extend the elbow, and rotate the forearm both inwards and outwards.

A Word of Advice > Strength sports and similar activities, in which weights and other objects are held tightly, can lead to further irritation of the affected muscles and should therefore be avoided.

Forearm fascia

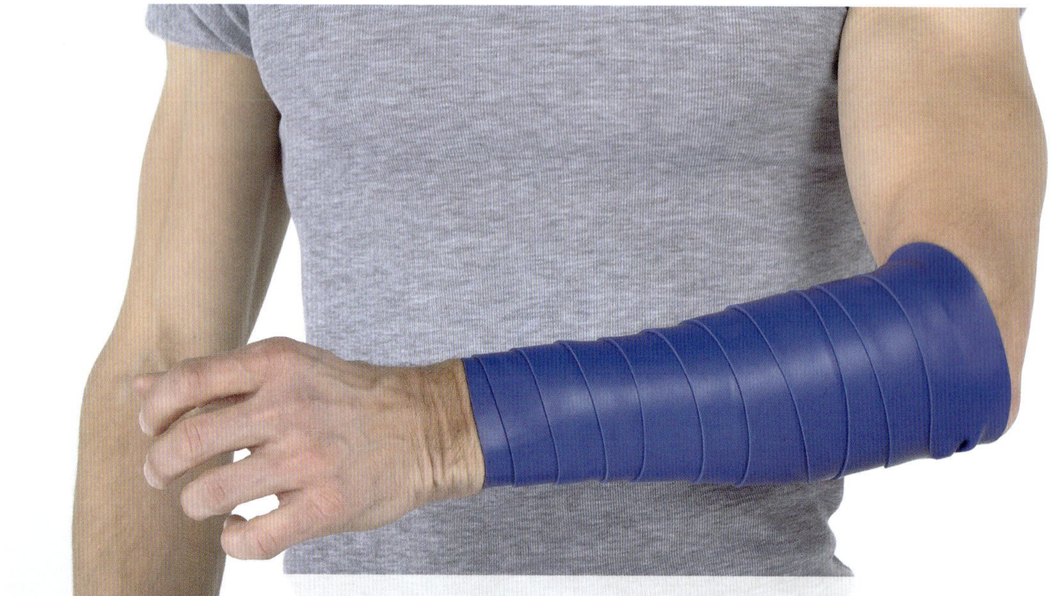

Painful region: the forearm fascia

Adhesions involving the upper arm fascia can lead to pain in various regions of the forearm, depending on which part of the fascia is affected. Pain is often felt during supination and pronation. This also determines the technique used to apply the flossing band wrap.

The flossing band wrap ⇢ Here's how it works

1 The patient's elbow joint is slightly extended. Wind the first turn with 50% tension to anchor the band around the lower part of the forearm close to the wrist.

2 Now wind the flossing band in ascending circular turns. The band should overlap 50% at each turn. A tension of 60–80% should be applied in the region of the adhesions and the painful fascia, with a tension of 50% on the other side of the forearm.

3 Using the same technique, wind the band up to the elbow joint and secure it into place.

Where it hurts on movement

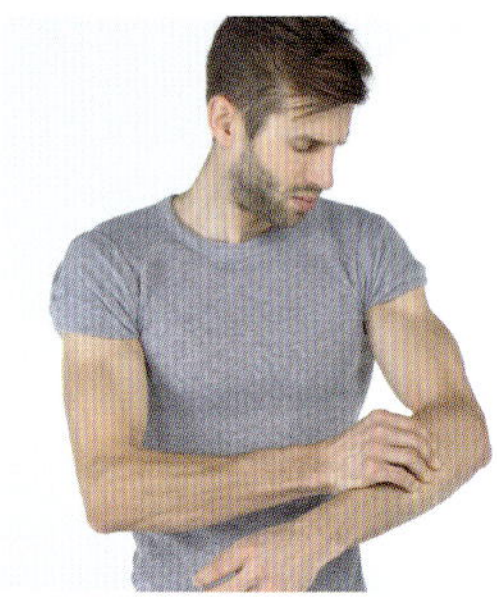

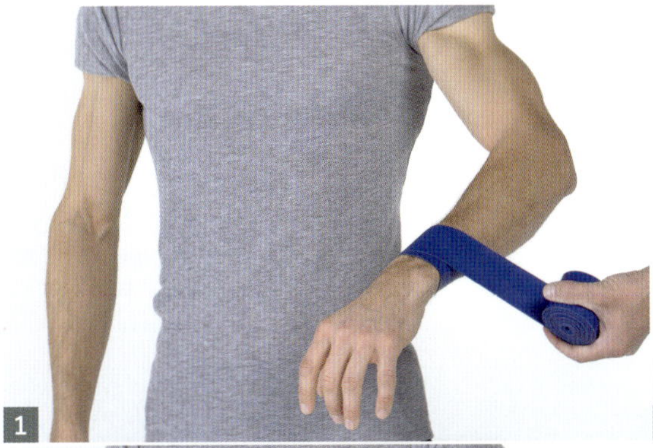
1

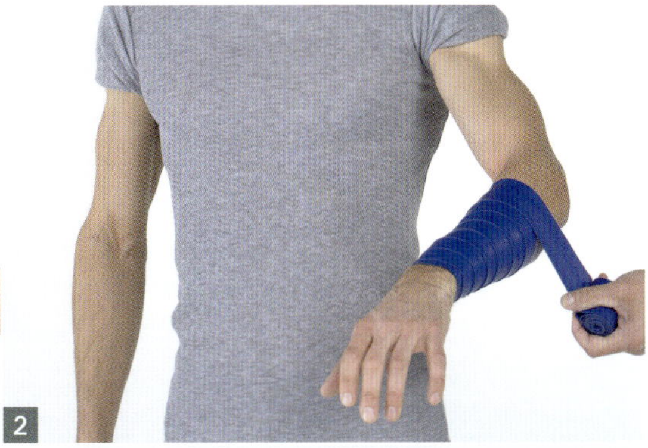
2

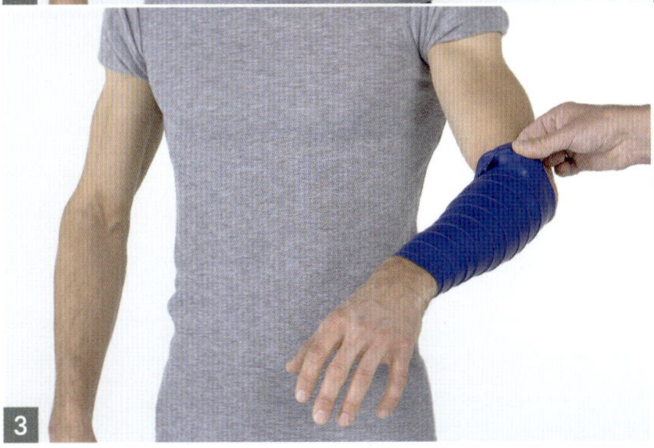
3

Material: Flossing band
Length: 2.06 m
Width: 5 cm
Tension: Painful region 60–80%, other side 50%

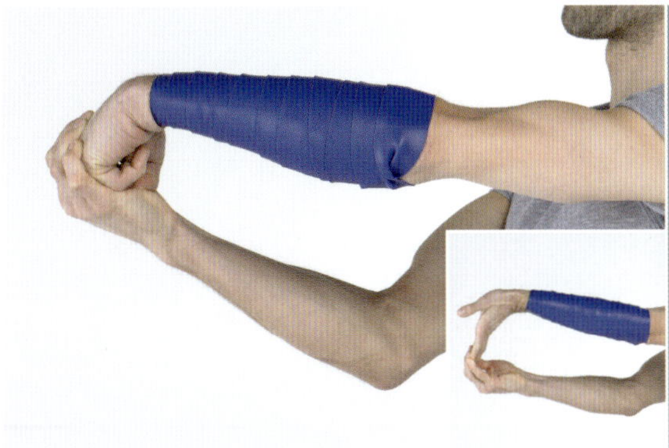

Active Exercise

Flex the fingers and wrist joint maximally. After this, extend the fingers and the wrist joint maximally. Finally, perform maximal inward and outward rotational movements with your forearm.

A Word of Advice > If there is pain in the muscles of the forearm and hand, strength sports as well as intensive lifting and carrying should be avoided.

Wrist joint

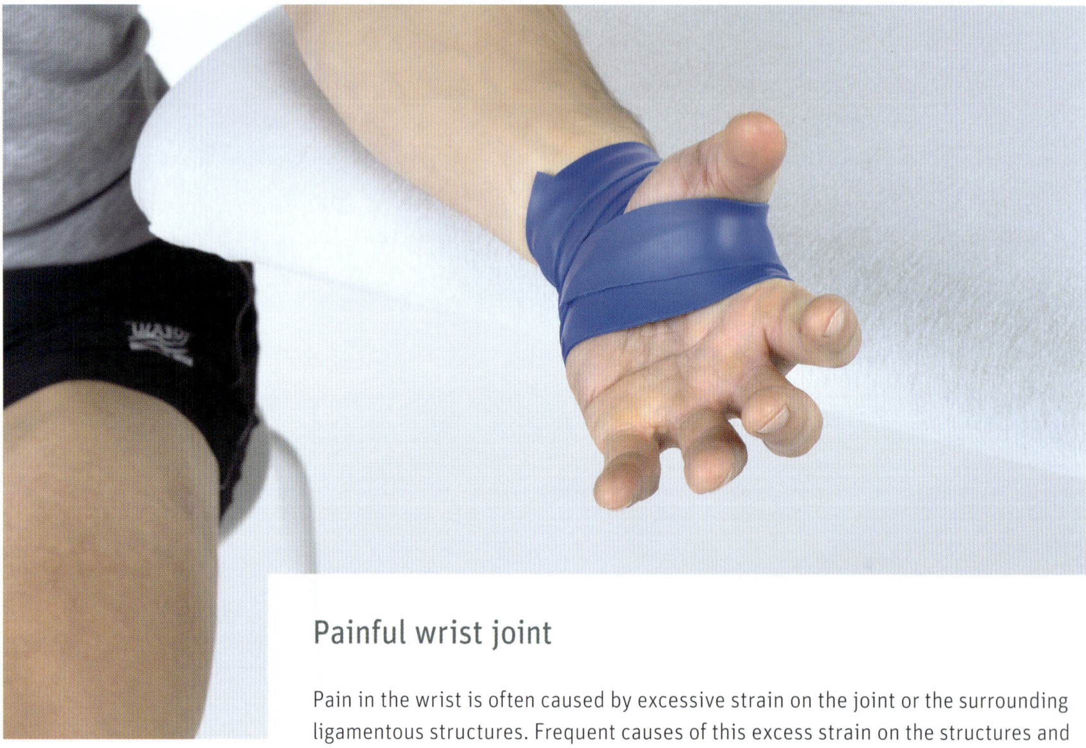

Painful wrist joint

Pain in the wrist is often caused by excessive strain on the joint or the surrounding ligamentous structures. Frequent causes of this excess strain on the structures and of the pain include a direct fall onto the hand (outstretched for support) or a force which causes the wrist to bend back sharply.

The flossing band wrap ⇢ Here's how it works

1 The patient's elbow is supported on the therapy couch. The wrist is bent back slightly. Wind the first turn with 50% tension to anchor the band around the metacarpal bones.

2 Now wind the flossing band in a figure-of-eight turn, first around the wrist and then back around the hand. Continue these figure-of-eight turns around the hand and the joint. The band should overlap slightly at each turn. A tension of 60–80% should be applied over one side of the painful wrist joint, with a tension of 50% on the other side and on the hand.

3 Using the same technique, keep winding the band up to its end and secure it into place.

Painful movement

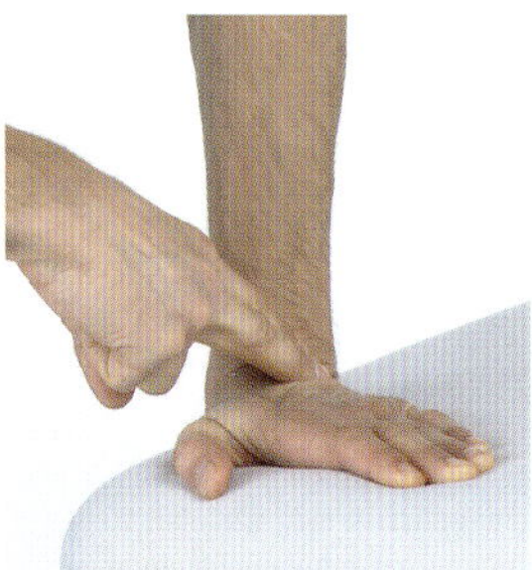

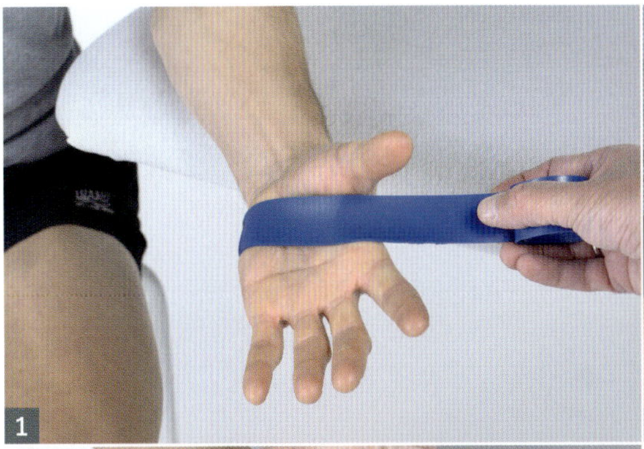

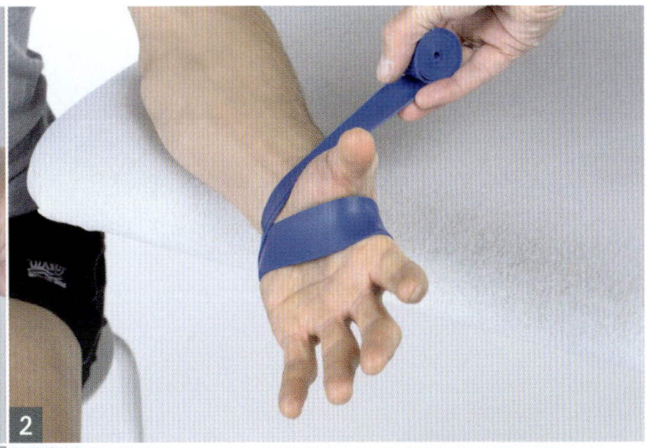

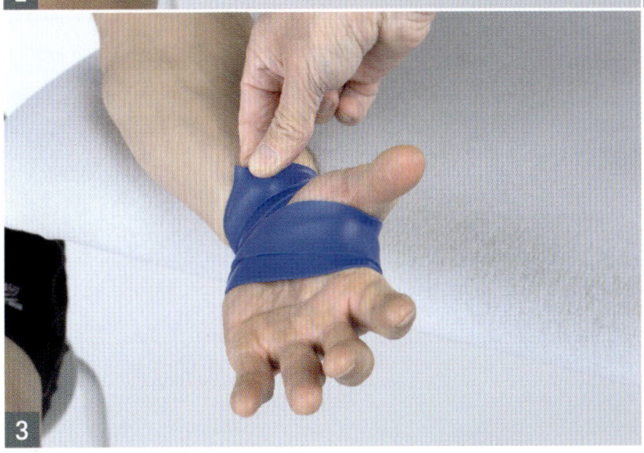

Material: Flossing band
Length: 1.03 m
Width: 2.5 cm
Tension: Painful region 60–80%, other side and hand 50%

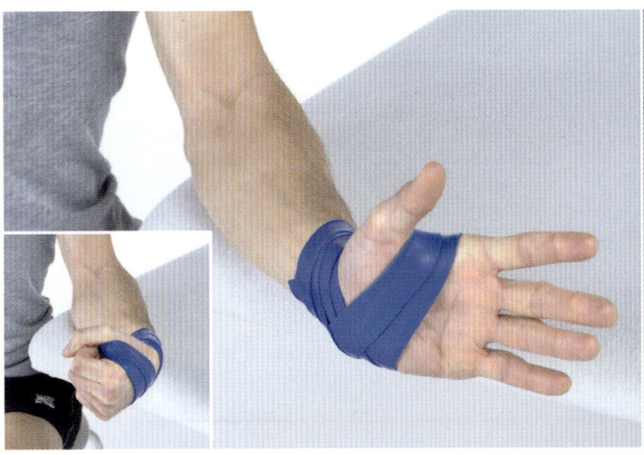

Active Exercise

Extend the fingers and the wrist joint maximally, then flex the fingers and the wrist joint maximally. After this, bend the wrist sideways to the thumb side and to the little finger side.

A Word of Advice > If numbness of the fingers occurs, the flossing band should not be applied quite so tightly to the forearm. Pain in the wrist joint can occur in racket sports and strength training, if the joint is not sufficiently well stabilized.

Finger joints, collateral ligaments

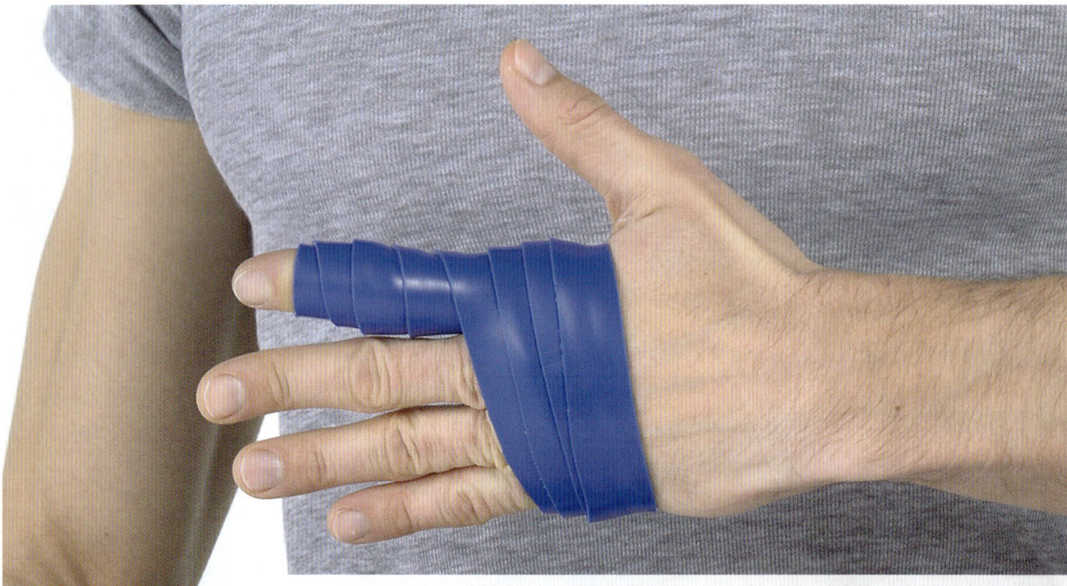

Painful finger joints, collateral ligaments

In most cases, pain in the finger joints occurs when the ligamentous structures of the joints are overstretched. This may happen as a result of a fall or the action of any other force on the finger (e.g. the impact of a ball on the fingertip).

The flossing band wrap ⇢ Here's how it works

1 The patient's fingers are spread out and the affected finger is extended. Wind the first turn with 50% tension to anchor the band around the tip of the finger.

2 Now wind the flossing band in ascending circular turns. The band should overlap 50% at each turn. A tension of 60–80% should be applied in the region of the affected collateral ligaments, with a tension of 50% on the other side of the finger.

3 Using the same technique, wind the band up to the palm of the hand; the last turn should be wound around the metacarpus and secured into place there.

Where it hurts on movement

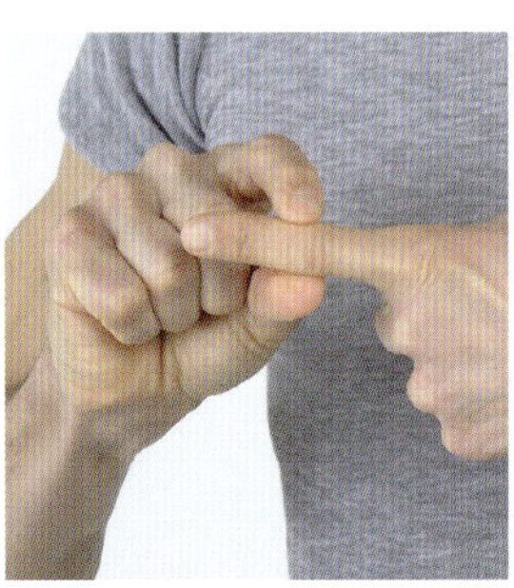

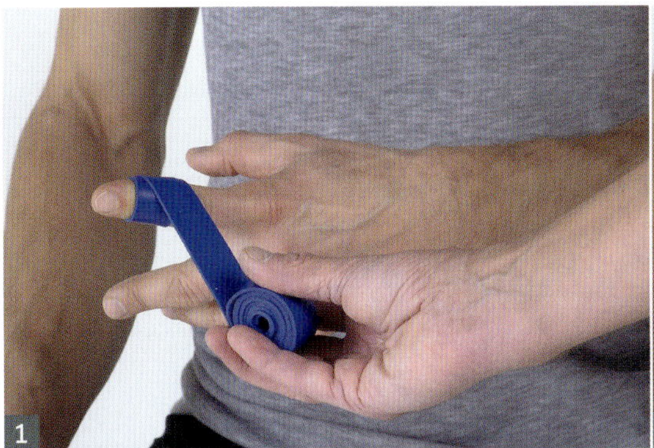

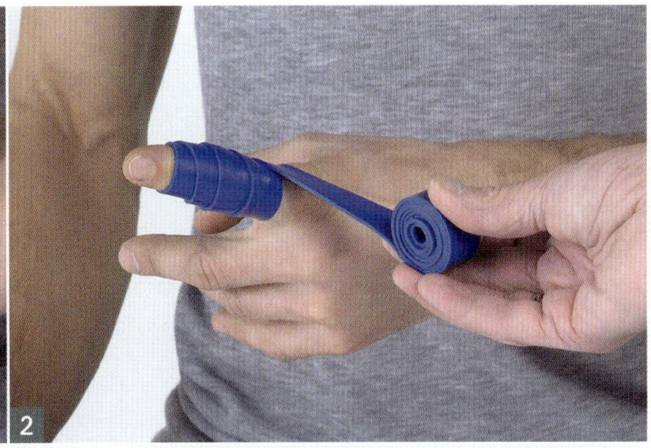

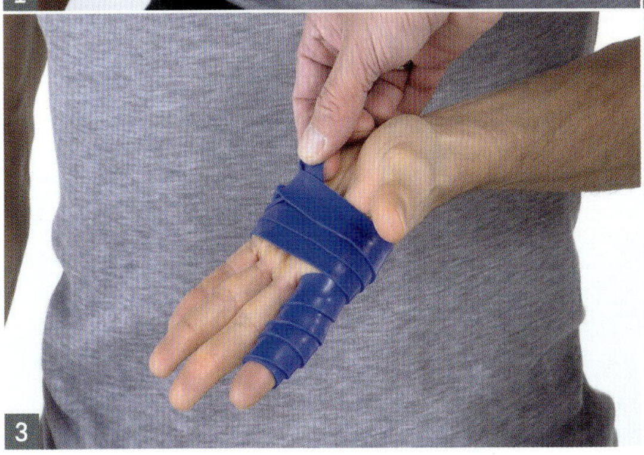

Material: Flossing band
Length: 1.03 m
Width: 2.5 cm
Tension: Painful region 60–80%, other side 50%

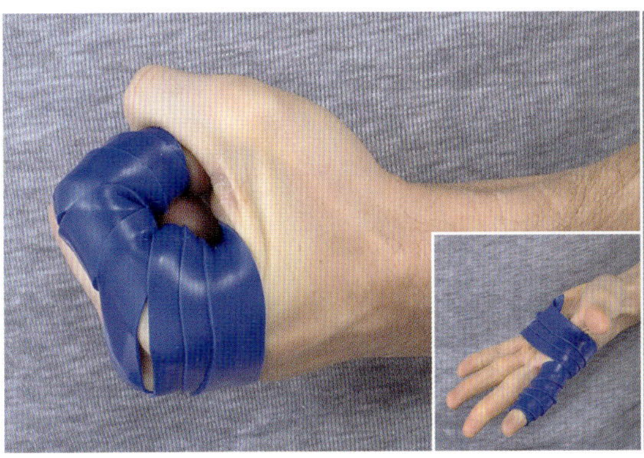

Active Exercise

Extend and flex the affected finger maximally. As an alternative, you could also grasp a sponge rubber ball (or a similar object), squeeze it tightly, and then let go again.

A Word of Advice > Finger injuries are very painful. Do not resume sports activities too soon! Frontal impact on the fingers should be avoided (e.g. volleyball, basketball, handball).

Thumb joints

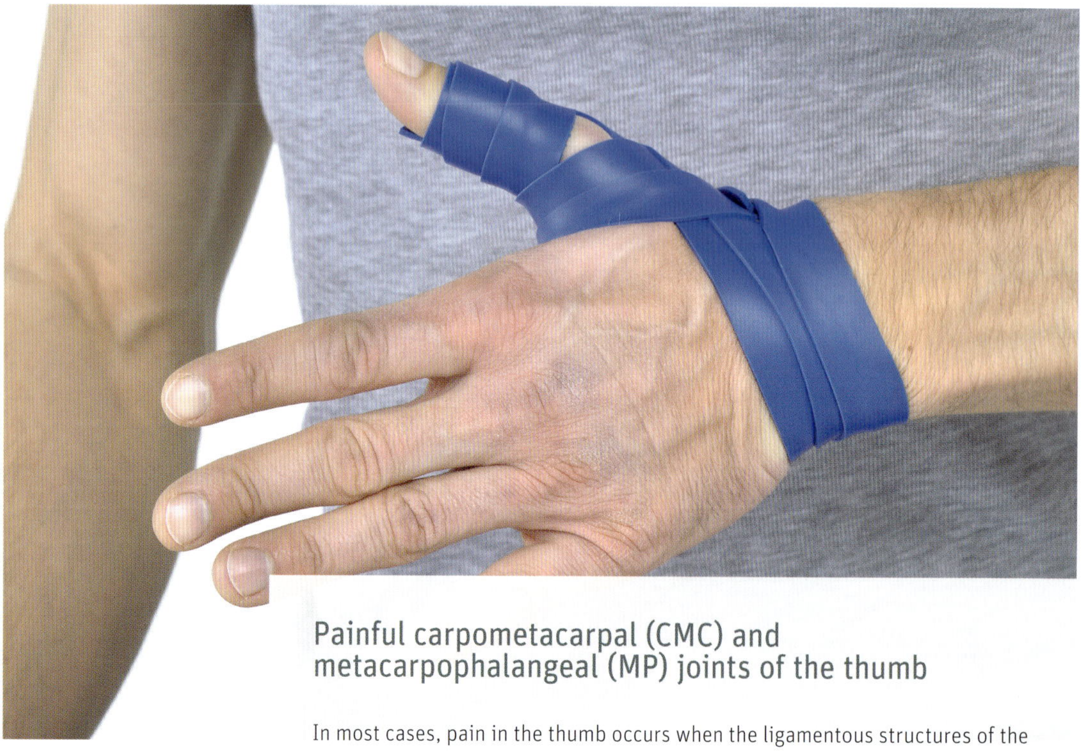

Painful carpometacarpal (CMC) and metacarpophalangeal (MP) joints of the thumb

In most cases, pain in the thumb occurs when the ligamentous structures of the joints are overstretched. This may happen as a result of a fall onto the thumb or the action of any other force on it, e.g. during skiing due to leverage from the ski pole loop (skier's thumb), or from the impact of a ball on the tip of the thumb.

The flossing band wrap → Here's how it works

1 The patient's fingers are spread out and the thumb is extended. Wind the first turn with 50% tension to anchor the band around the thumb.

2 Now wind the flossing band in a figure-of-eight turn around the affected joint and around the wrist. A tension of 60–80% should be applied in the region of the affected joint, with a tension of 50% elsewhere.

3 Continue winding the band in figure-of-eight turns around the thumb joint and the wrist; the last turn is wound around the wrist and secured into place there.

Where it hurts on movement

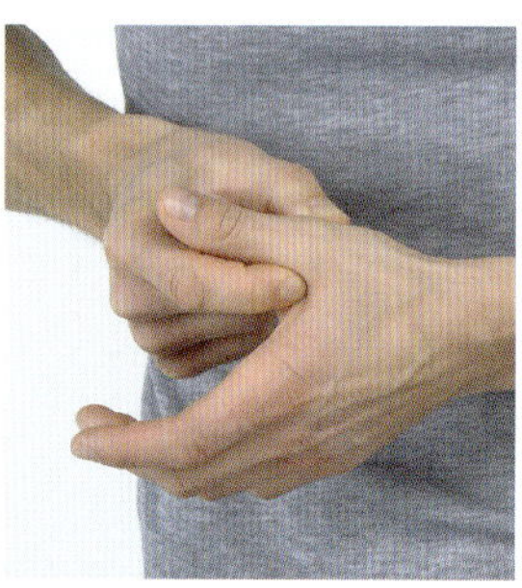

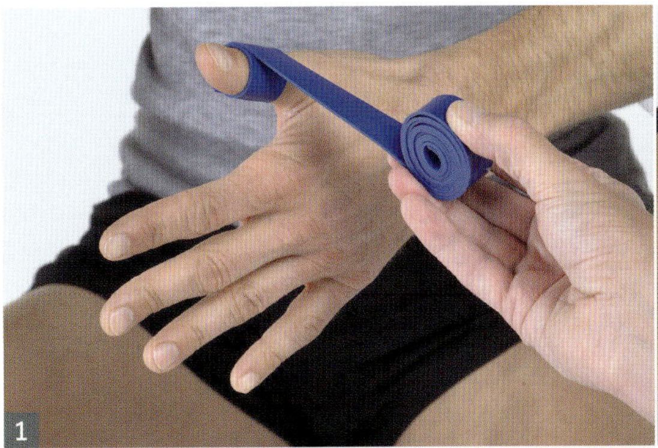

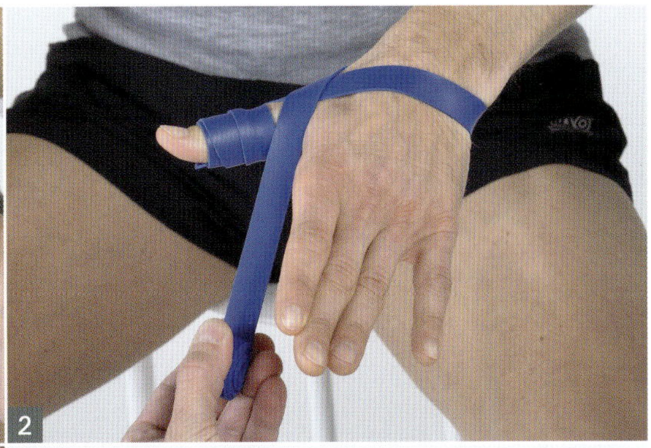

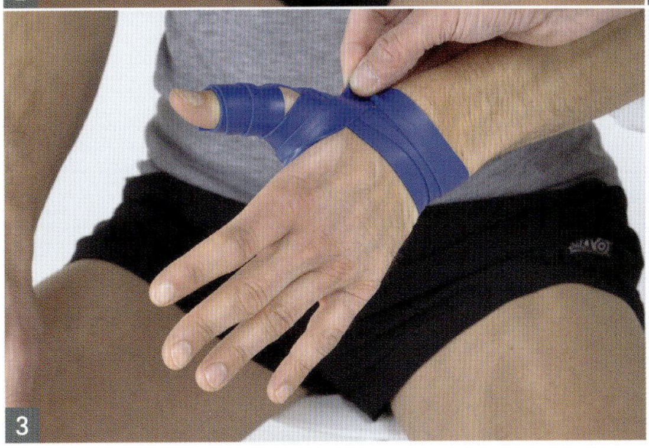

Material: Flossing band
Length: 1.03 m
Width: 2.5 cm
Tension: Painful region 60–80%, otherwise 50%

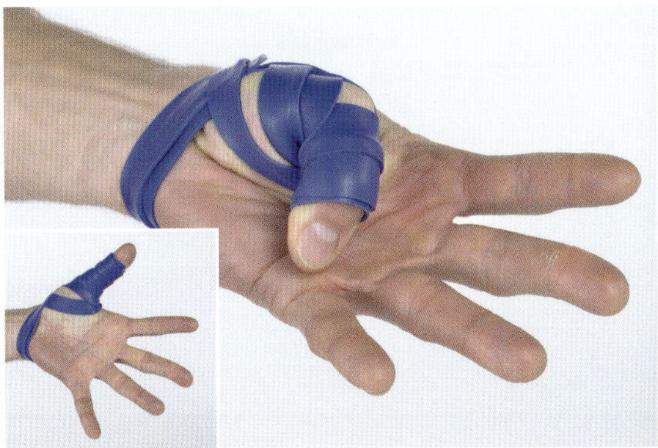

Active Exercise

Extend and flex the thumb maximally. Bring the thumb to each of its opposing fingers or close the fingers over the thumb. Flex and extend the wrist joint.

A Word of Advice > Frontal impact on the thumb should be avoided (e.g. volleyball, basketball, handball). If the action of an external force on the thumb has caused severe pain, consult a doctor to rule out a bone fracture.

Upper arm swellings

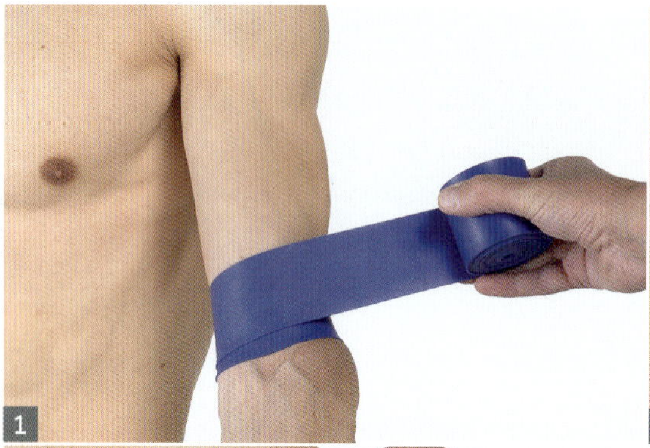

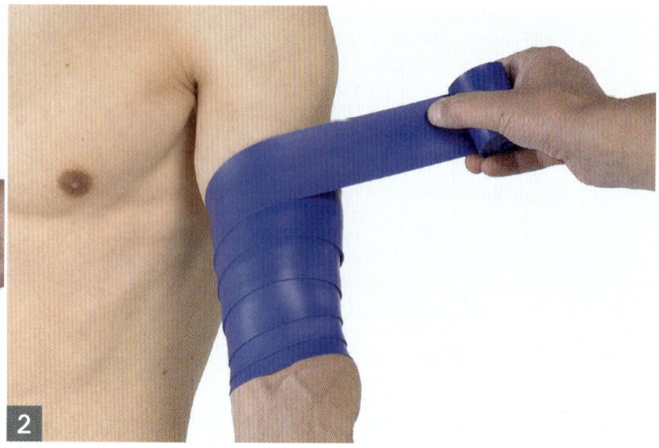

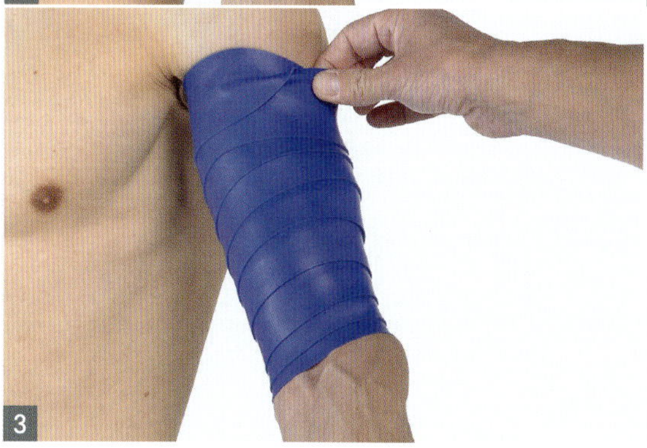

Material: Flossing band
Length: 2.06 m
Width: 5 cm
Tension: 50% overall

Upper arm swellings

Swellings of the upper arm frequently occur following injuries to the shoulder and upper arm, and also following surgery to the female breast. A swelling indicates that the tissue fluid cannot drain away quickly enough.

The Flossing band wrap → Here's how it works

1 The patient's arm is extended, with the hand supported on the therapy couch. Wind the first turn with 50% tension to anchor the band below the swelling on the upper arm.

2 Now wind the flossing band in ascending circular turns. The band should overlap 50% each time. A tension of 50% should be applied over the entire swollen region.

3 Using the same technique, wind the band around the whole swelling towards the shoulder in proximal direction and secure it into place.

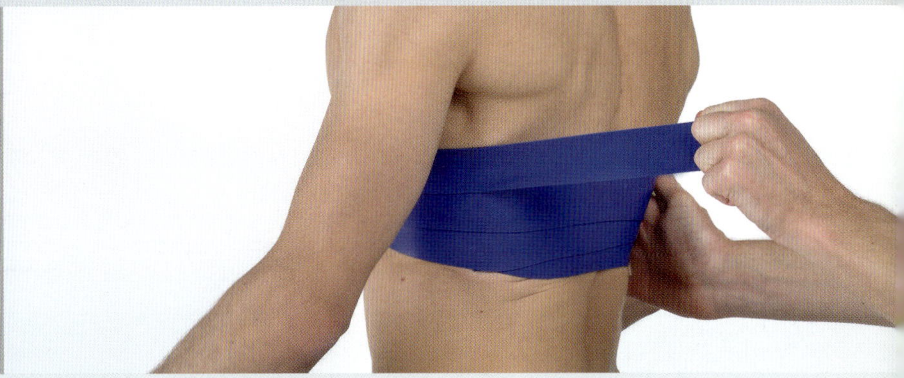

Chapter 2: Flossing Band Wraps for Abdominal and Back Pain

Thoracic spine

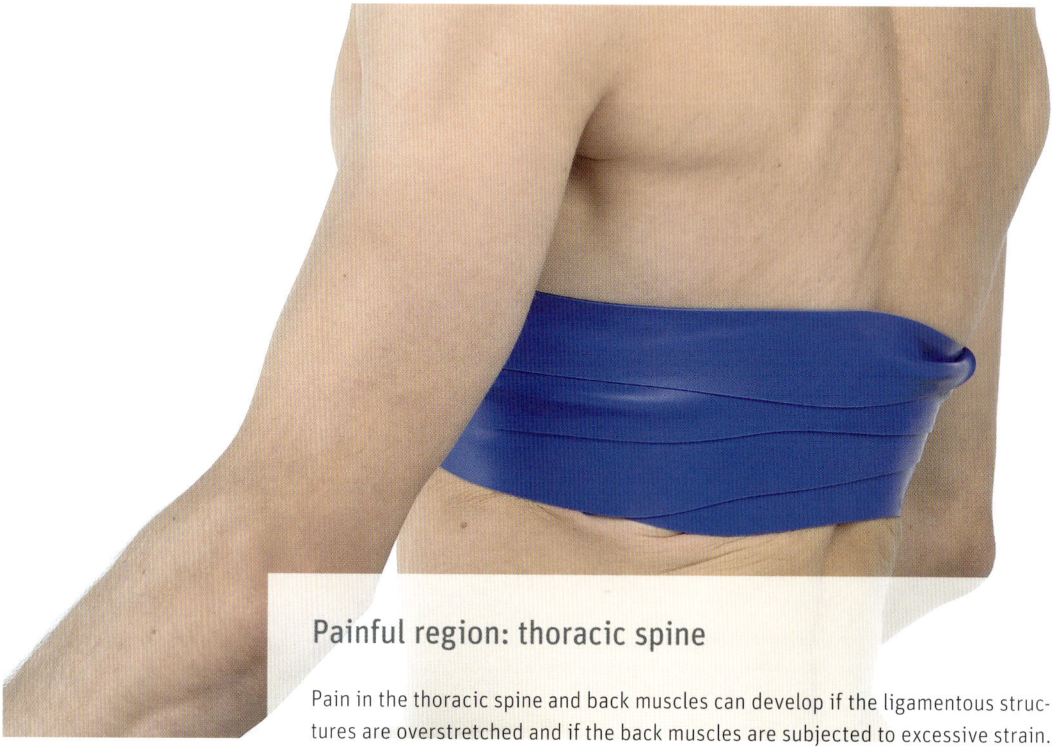

Painful region: thoracic spine

Pain in the thoracic spine and back muscles can develop if the ligamentous structures are overstretched and if the back muscles are subjected to excessive strain. Muscle tension often occurs for postural reasons (slouching) or following heavy physical exertion.

The flossing band wrap ⇢ Here's how it works

1 The patient should sit up as straight as possible. Wind the first turn with 50% tension to anchor the band around the thorax, just below the most painful region.

2 Now wind the flossing band around the thorax in ascending circular turns. The band should overlap 50% at each turn. A tension of 60–80% should be applied over the most painful part of the thoracic spine, with 50% tension over the anterior side of the thorax.

3 Using the same technique, wind the band to the end and secure it into place.

Painful movement

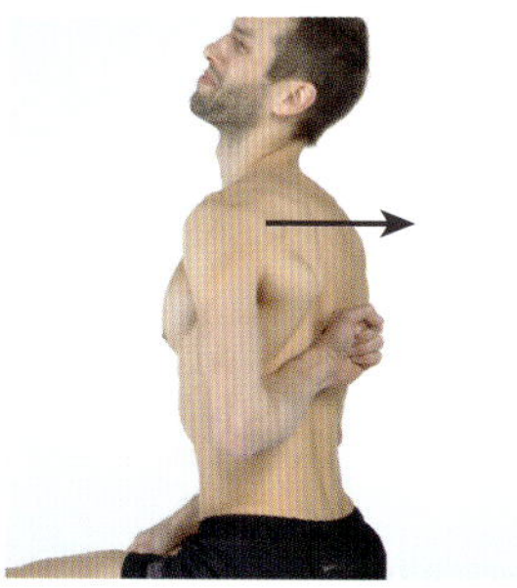

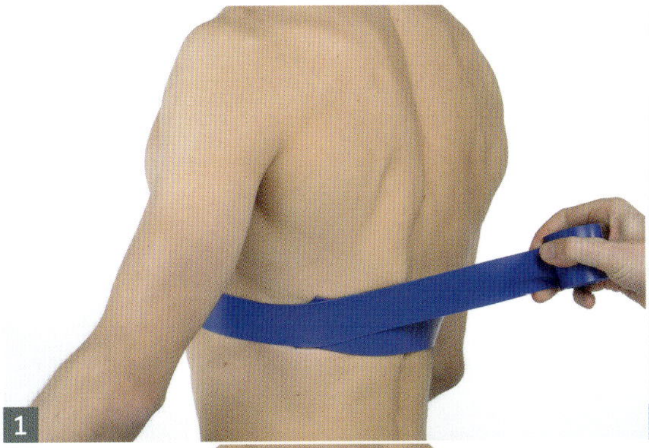
1

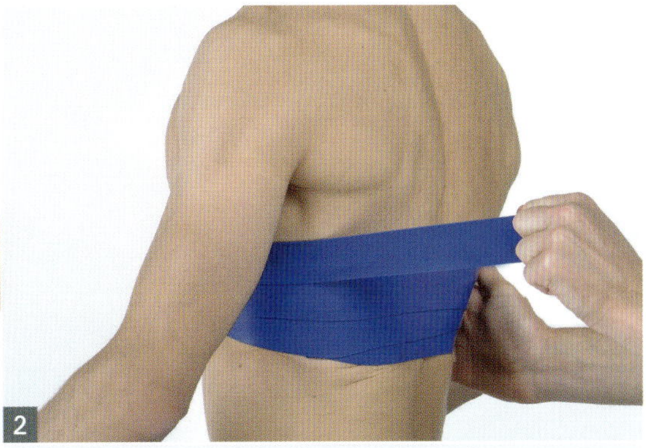
2

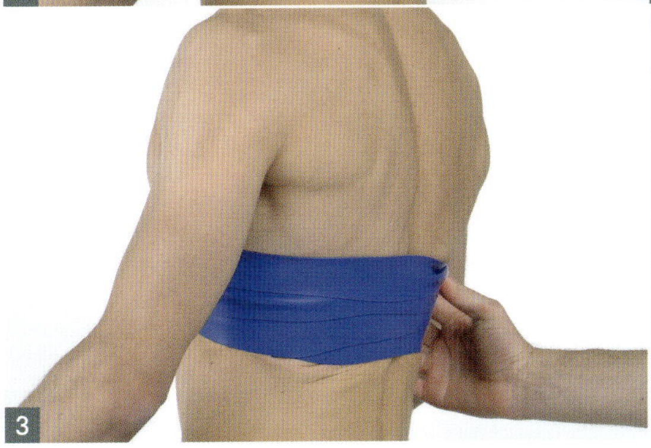
3

Material: Flossing band
Length: 2.06 m
Width: 5 cm
Tension: back 60–80%, front 50%

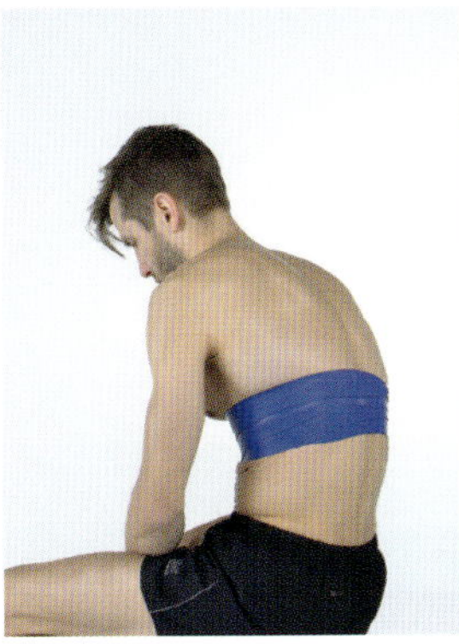

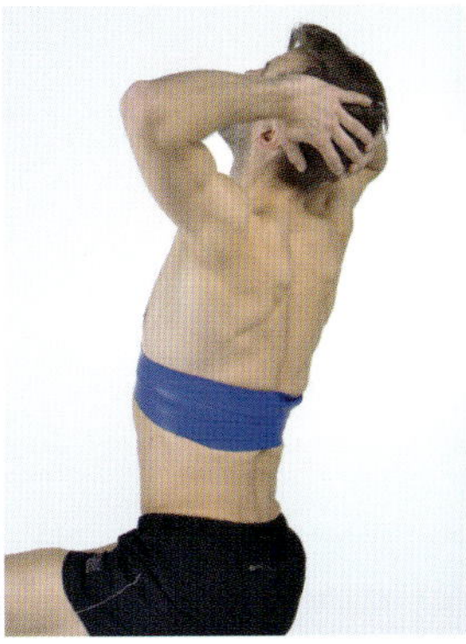

Active Exercise

Flex and extend the thoracic spine as best you can; the alternative is to rotate the torso to the right and left and perform lateral bends to both sides. In addition, you can breathe in and out deeply during the movement, and also move the arms along.

A Word of Advice > Walking or swimming are particularly to be recommended for thoracic spine pain, as these forms of exercise encourage you to straighten your body and to move and stretch the spine uniformly.

Ribs/breathing

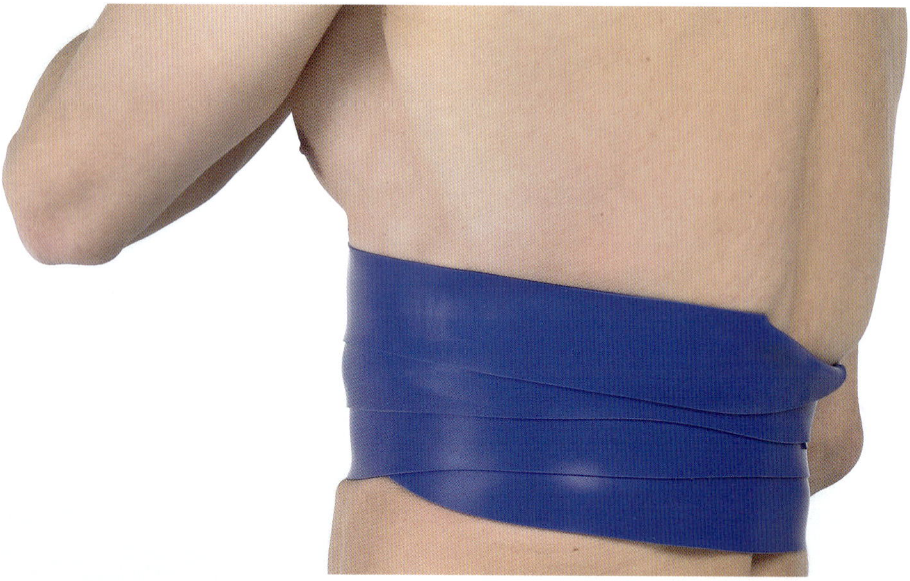

Painful region: ribs/breathing

Pain in the ribs is usually due to the action of a direct force on the thorax. Examples of this include slipping on ice, a fall at home, a bicycling accident or a sports-related fall. Since the ribs move with every breath, rib injuries are very painful and often heal slowly. The bones are usually compressed and the muscles torn or sprained.

The flossing band wrap ⇢ Here's how it works

1 The patient should sit up or stand as straight as possible. Wind the first turn with 50% tension to anchor the band around the thorax below the most painful region.

2 Now wind the flossing band around the thorax in ascending circular turns. The band should overlap 50% at each turn. A tension of 60–80% should be applied to the most painful region, with 50% tension over the other side of the thorax.

3 Using the same technique, wind the band to the end and secure it into place.

Where it hurts on movement

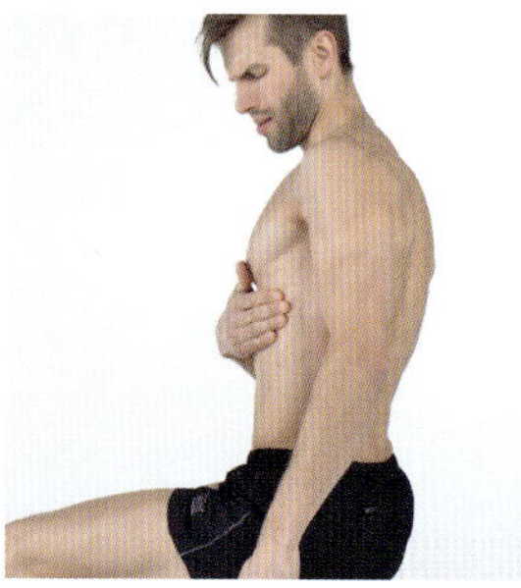

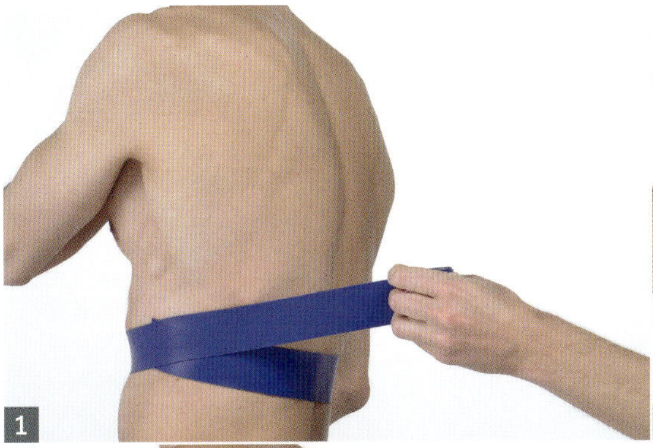
1

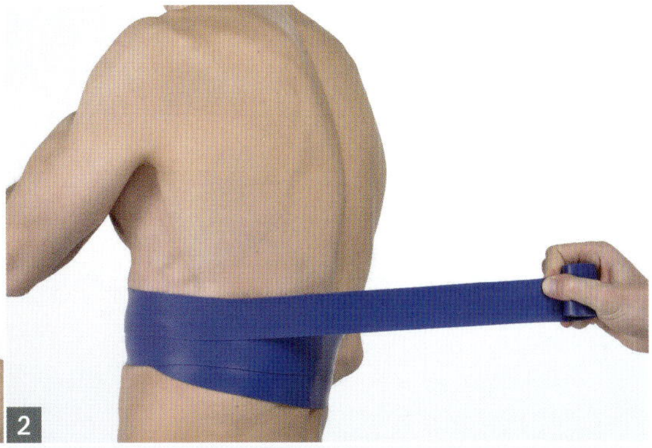
2

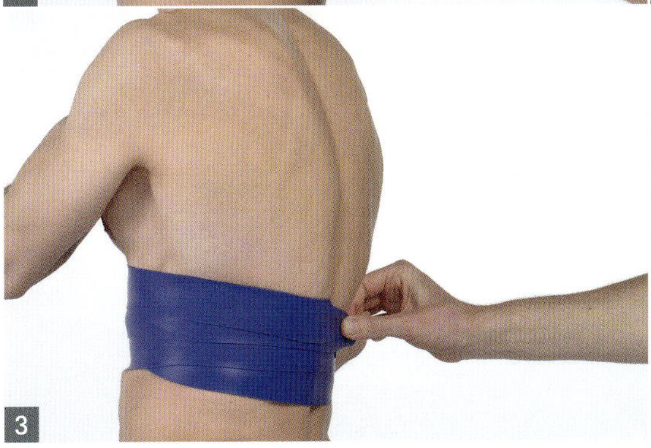
3

Material: Flossing band
Length: 2.06 m
Width: 5 cm
Tension: Painful region 60-80%, other side 50%

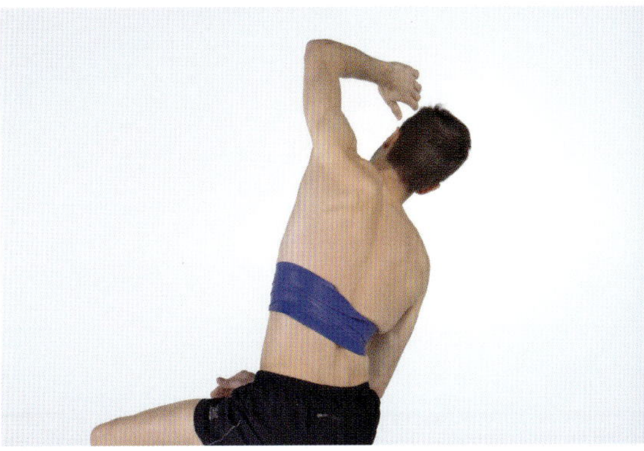

Active Exercise

Sit or stand upright, extend the arm on the affected side up over the head and bend to the opposite side. Breathe in and out deeply several times. In addition, you should flex and extend the whole spine, and also rotate (twist) it to both sides.

A Word of Advice > Avoid compensatory postures or prolonged inactivity, since the lungs need to be well-ventilated to prevent pulmonary disease (pneumonia etc.).
If this winding method is too painful for the patient, the wrap can also be applied with less tension.

Lumbar spine

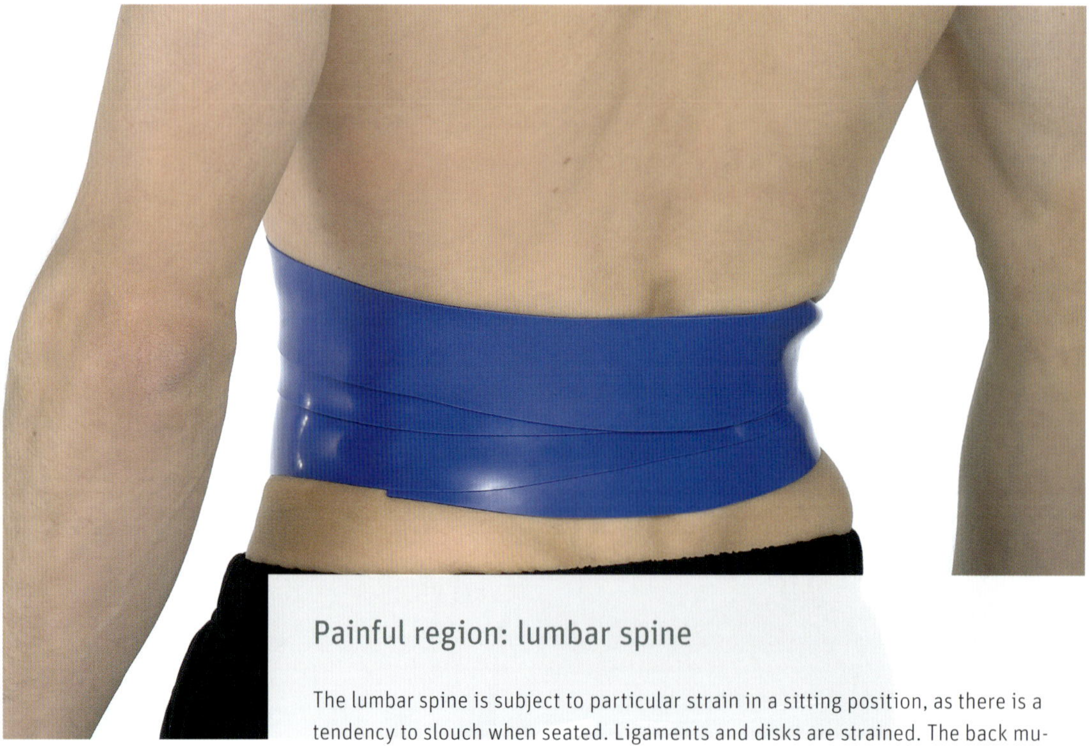

Painful region: lumbar spine

The lumbar spine is subject to particular strain in a sitting position, as there is a tendency to slouch when seated. Ligaments and disks are strained. The back muscles try to counteract this strain and tense up. Of course, pain in the lumbar spine and back muscles can also develop following heavy physical exertion.

The flossing band wrap ⟶ Here's how it works

1 The patient should sit up or stand as straight as possible. Wind the first turn with 50% tension to anchor the band around the back and abdomen below the painful region.

2 Now wind the flossing band around the torso in ascending circular turns. The band should overlap 50% at each turn. A tension of 60–80% should be applied over the most painful part of the lumbar spine, with 50% tension applied to the other side (abdomen).

3 Using the same technique, wind the band to the end and secure it into place.

Painful movement

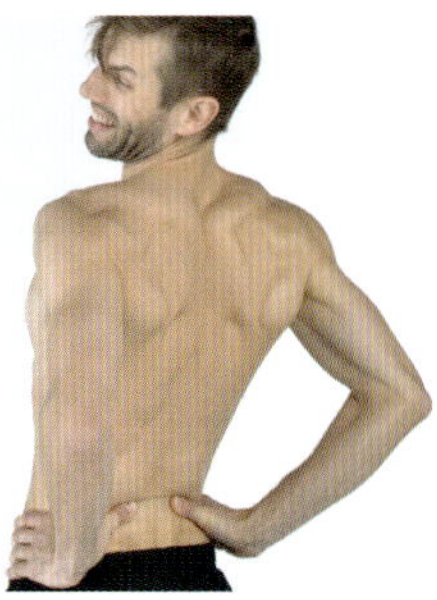

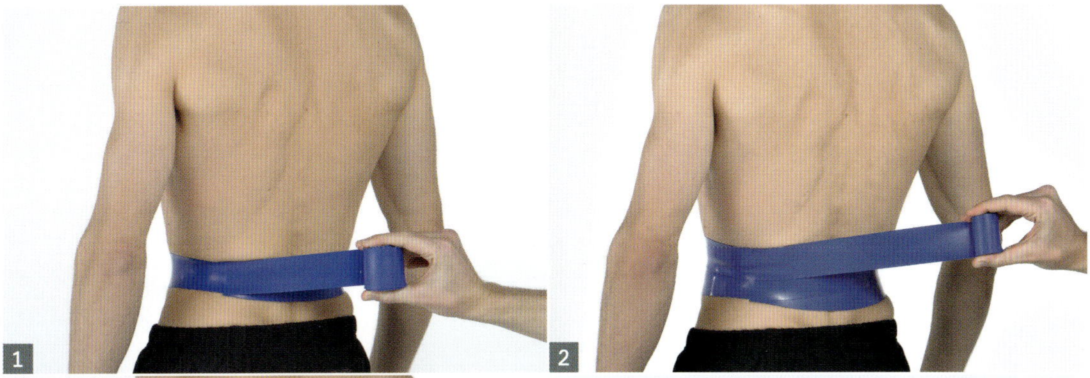

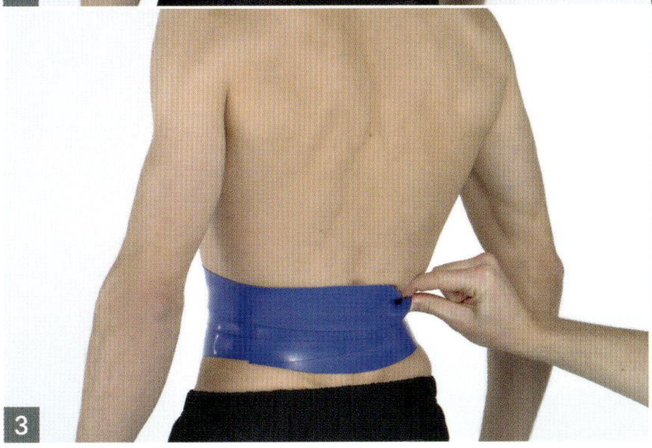

Material: Flossing band
Length: 2.06 m
Width: 5 cm
Tension: back 60–80%, front 50%

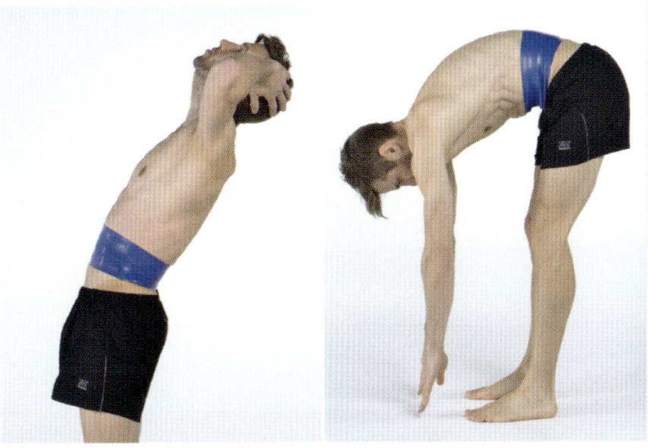

Active Exercise

Stand upright and do a deep forward bend; as an alternative, perform rotatory movements (twists) and lateral bends of the torso to both sides. The movements of the spine should also be combined with arm and leg stretches. For example, you could move your elbow towards the opposite knee.

A Word of Advice > If the pain spreads and if numbness or paralysis develops, consult a doctor to rule out a disc prolapse!

Sacroiliac joints, symphysis

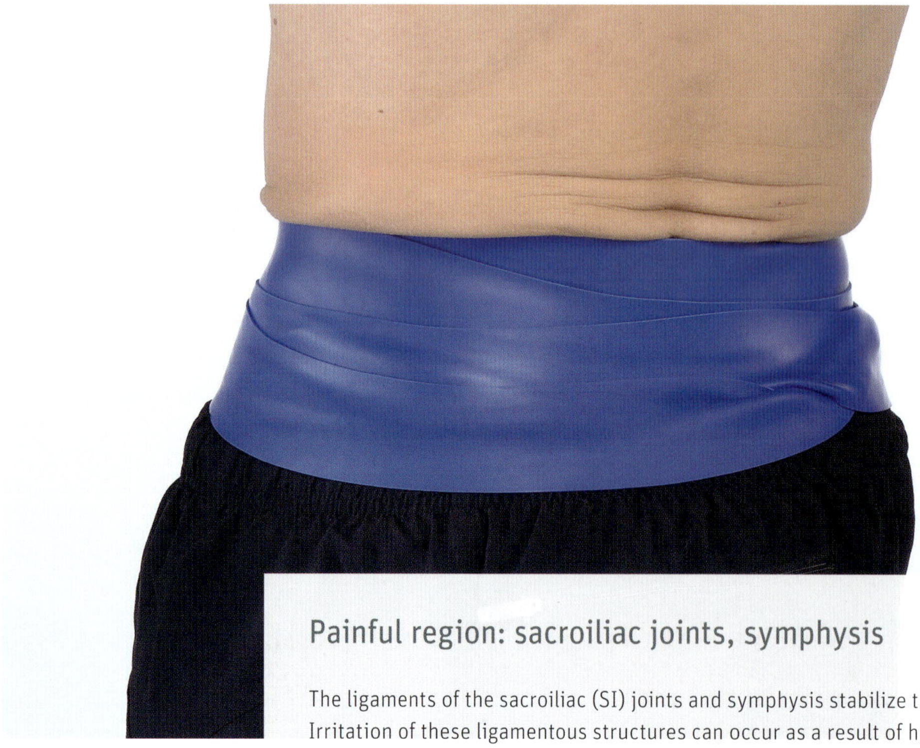

Painful region: sacroiliac joints, symphysis

The ligaments of the sacroiliac (SI) joints and symphysis stabilize the pelvis. Irritation of these ligamentous structures can occur as a result of heavy physical exertion or after a prolonged period in a slouched posture. A direct fall onto the buttocks or hormonal changes (pregnancy) can also lead to injury or loosening of the ligaments, which can be associated with pain.

The flossing band wrap → Here's how it works

1 The patient should sit up or stand as straight as possible. Wind the first turn with 50% tension to anchor the band around the pelvis below the wing of the ilium and the iliac spine.

2 Now wind the flossing band around the pelvis in descending circular turns. The band should overlap 50% at each turn. A tension of 60–80% should be applied in the sacroiliac region (or the symphysis, depending on the site of the pain), with 50% tension on the other side.

3 Using the same technique, wind the band to the end and secure it into place.

Where it hurts on movement

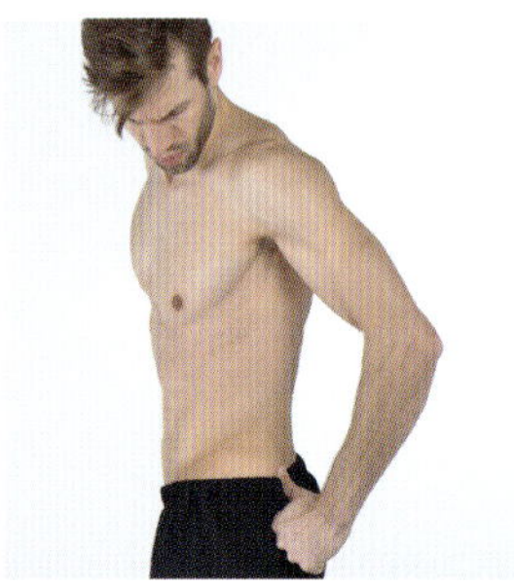

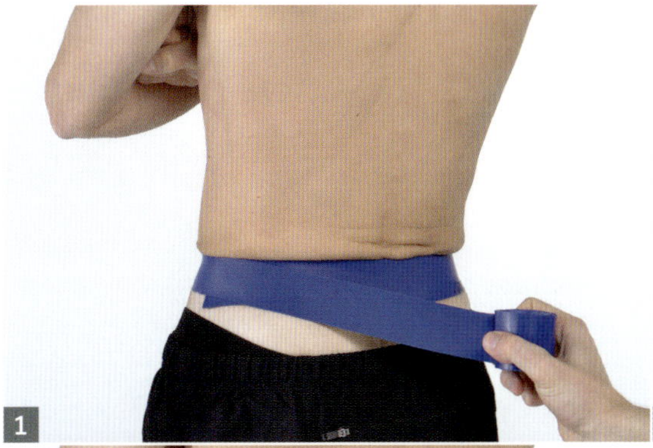

1

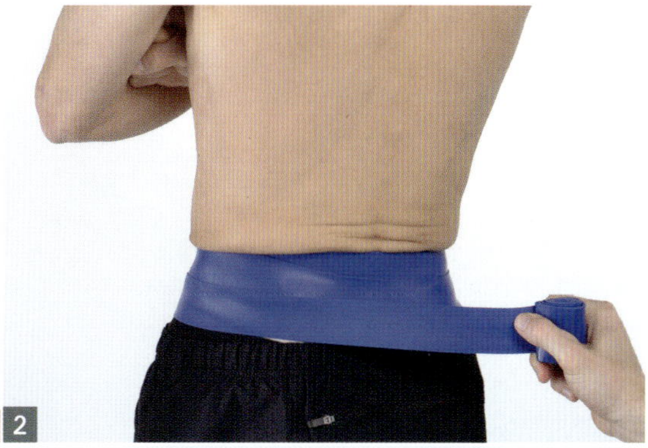

2

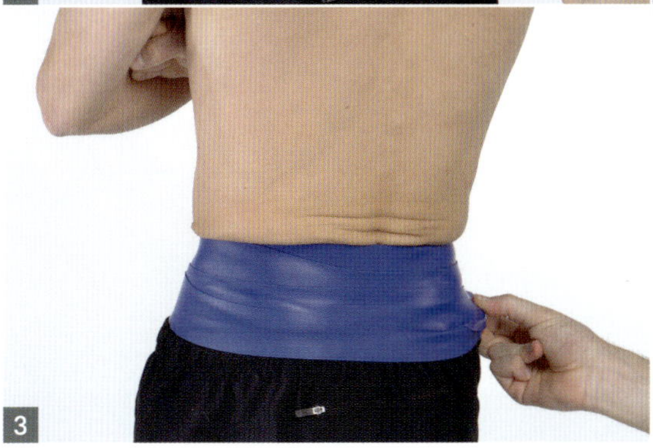

3

Material: Flossing band
Length: 2.06 m
Width: 5 cm
Tension: Painful region 60-80%, other side 50%

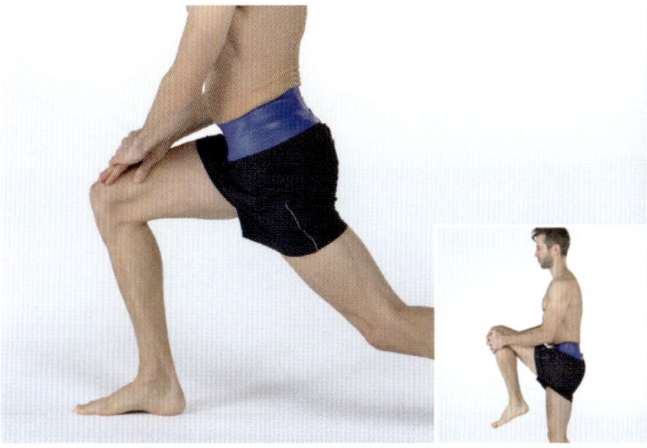

Active Exercise

Perform a wide reverse lunge and alternate this with flexing the hip joint as far as possible. By doing this, you will achieve forward and backward rotation in the SI joint. In addition, you could rotate (twist) the upper body to both sides, while keeping your feet in place.

A Word of Advice > A fall or jolt onto an extended leg (a "missed step"), may lead to severe irritation of the ligaments of the sacroiliac joint or symphysis.

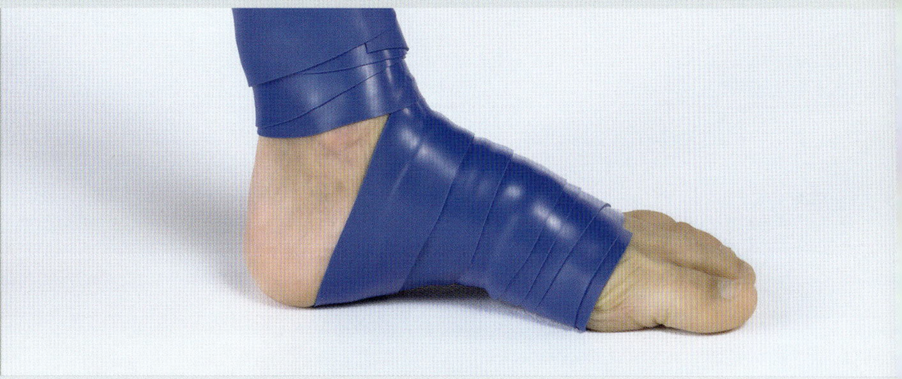

CHAPTER 3:
FLOSSING BAND WRAPS FOR LOWER EXTREMITY PAIN

Hip joint

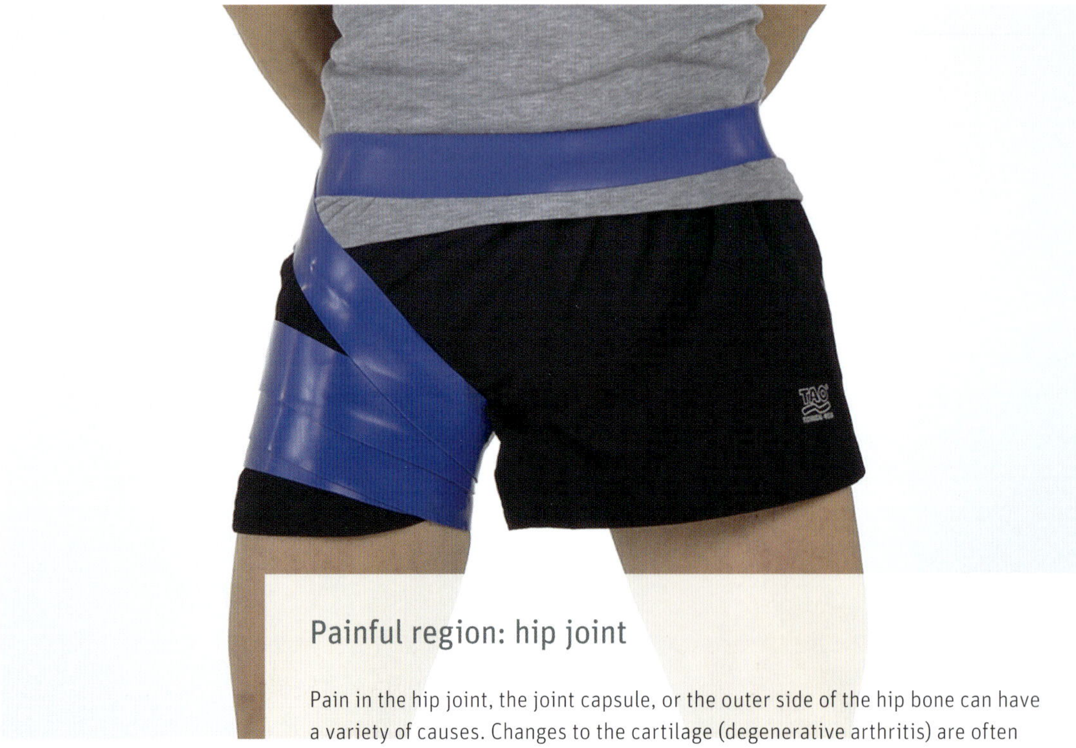

Painful region: hip joint

Pain in the hip joint, the joint capsule, or the outer side of the hip bone can have a variety of causes. Changes to the cartilage (degenerative arthritis) are often associated with pain deep in the groin. Other causes include overexertion during sports or at work, as well as being overweight. Pain at the outer hip bone is generally attributable to problems with the muscles that attach there. Long runs (jogging, etc.) – especially after periods of rest – can lead to severe irritation of the musculature surrounding the hip.

The flossing band wrap ⇢ Here's how it works

1 The patient stands with legs slightly apart. Wind the first turn with 50% tension to anchor the band around the upper part of the thigh.

Where it hurts on movement

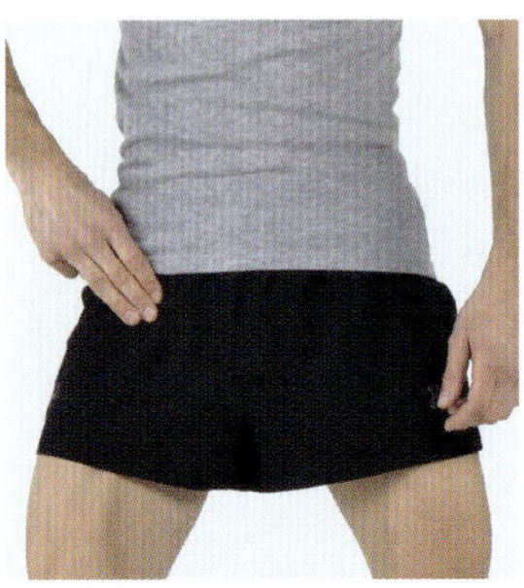

2 Now wind the flossing band around the thigh close to the groin, as far up as possible. A tension of 60–80% should be applied in the region of the hip joint and the lateral thigh (the trochanter major), with 50% tension on the inner side of the thigh.

3 A turn may be wound around the pelvis to stabilize the wrap. Secure the band into place at the pelvis.

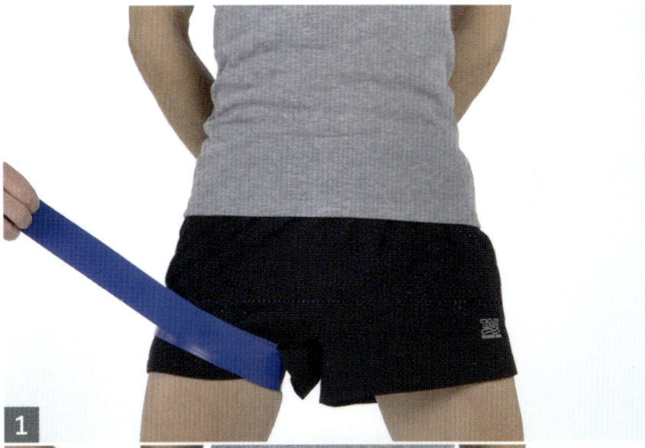

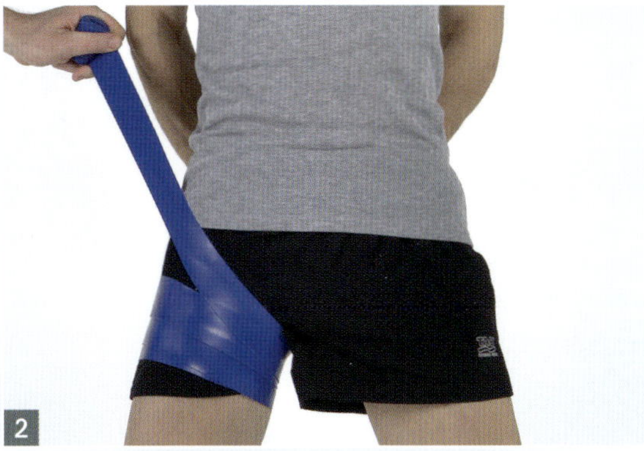

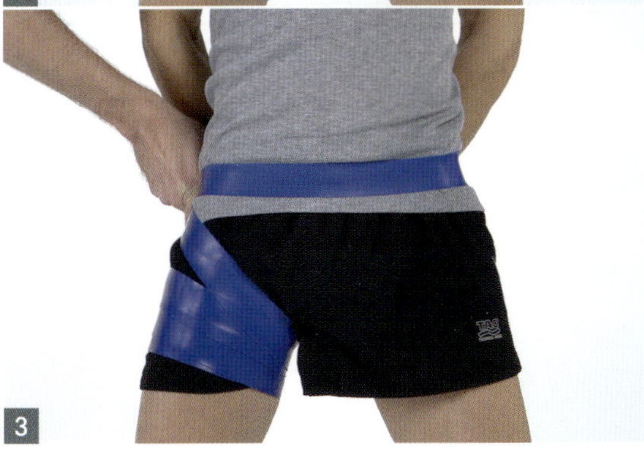

Material: Flossing band
Length: 2.06 m
Width: 5 cm
Tension: front/outside 60–80%, inside 50%

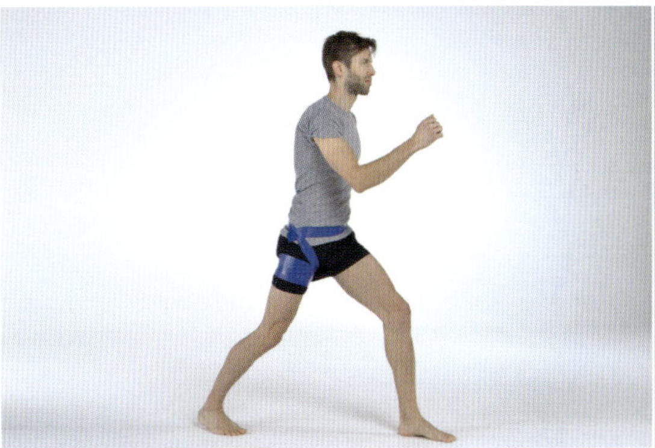

Active Exercise

Walk a few meters back and forth, taking big steps. You can also do knee bends or take big steps forwards and sideways, and then bend the knees gently.

A Word of Advice > Repeat these exercises several times, trying out all directions of movement while doing so. When the band is removed, the patient **must** lie down, as the rush of blood into the leg may cause dizziness!

Adductors

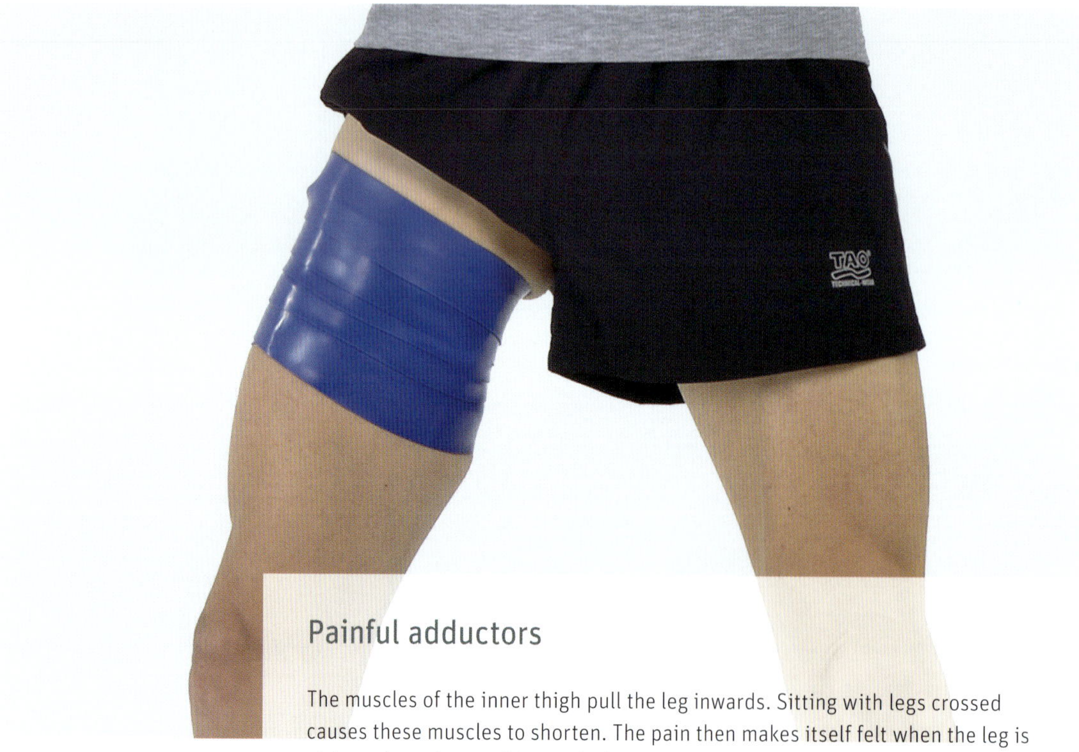

Painful adductors

The muscles of the inner thigh pull the leg inwards. Sitting with legs crossed causes these muscles to shorten. The pain then makes itself felt when the leg is abducted or when walking and playing sports. Intensive athletic activity or wide movements of the hip (straddle/sliding tackle, big sidestep, etc.) can also cause excessive strain on the adductors and a pulled muscle is a common result.

The flossing band wrap ⇢ Here's how it works

1 The patient stands with legs slightly apart. Wind the first turn with 50% tension to anchor the band around the upper part of the thigh.

2 Now wind the flossing band in ascending circular turns. The band should overlap 50% at each turn. Wind the band around the adductor region, as far as possible towards the groin. A tension of 60–80% should be applied over the adductors, with 50% tension on the outer (lateral) side of the thigh.

3 Using the same technique, wind the band as far up as possible and secure it into place.

Painful movement

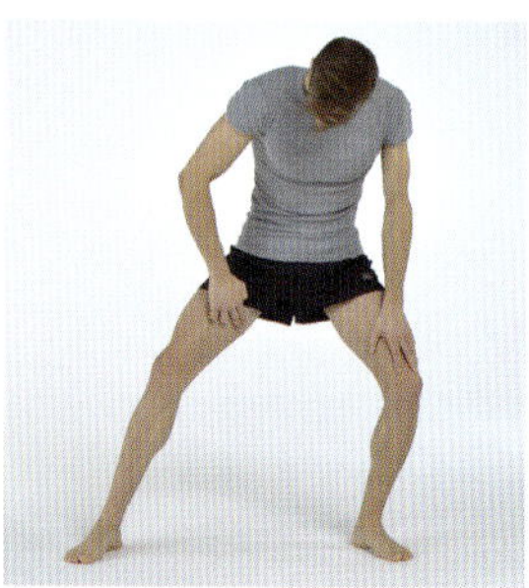

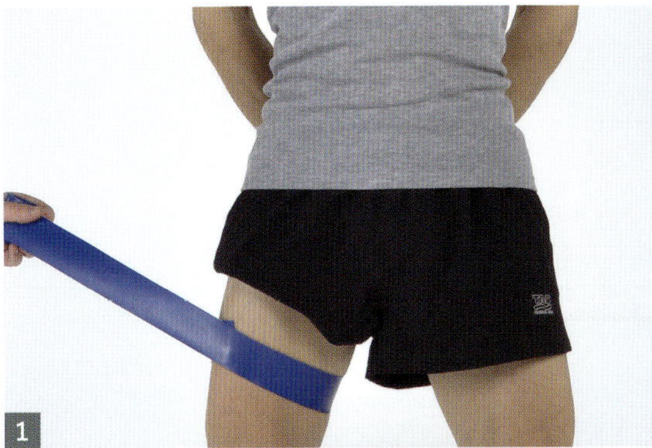

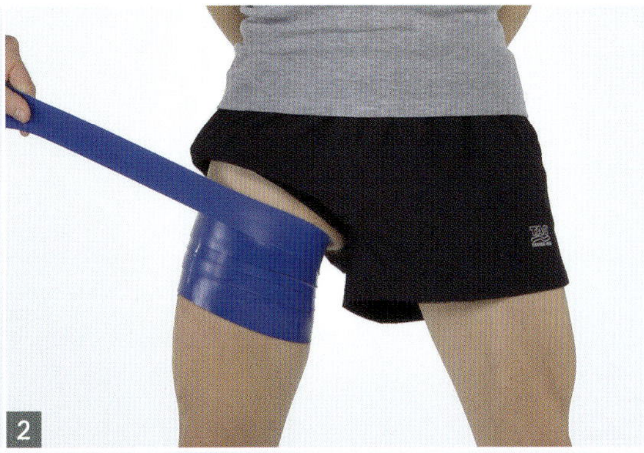

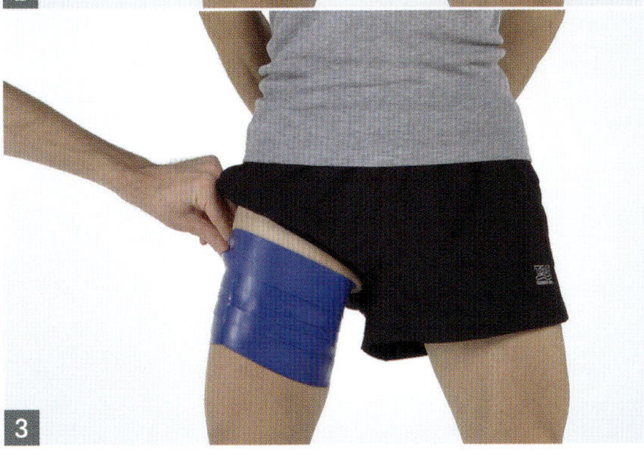

Material: Flossing band
Length: 2.06 m
Width: 5 cm
Tension: inside 60–80%, outside 50%

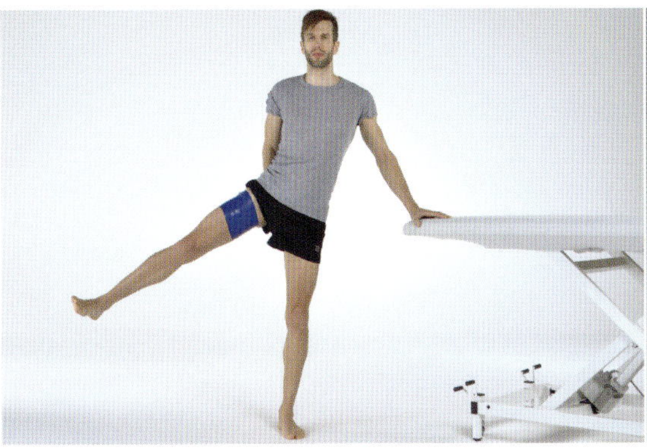

Active Exercise

While standing, abduct the leg and then bring it back again. The exercise can be made more dynamic by doing jumping jacks. But you can also just lie on your side and then abduct the leg towards the ceiling.

A Word of Advice > Repeat these exercises several times, trying out all directions of movement while doing so. When the band is removed, the patient **must** lie down, as the rush of blood into the leg may cause dizziness!

Lateral thigh

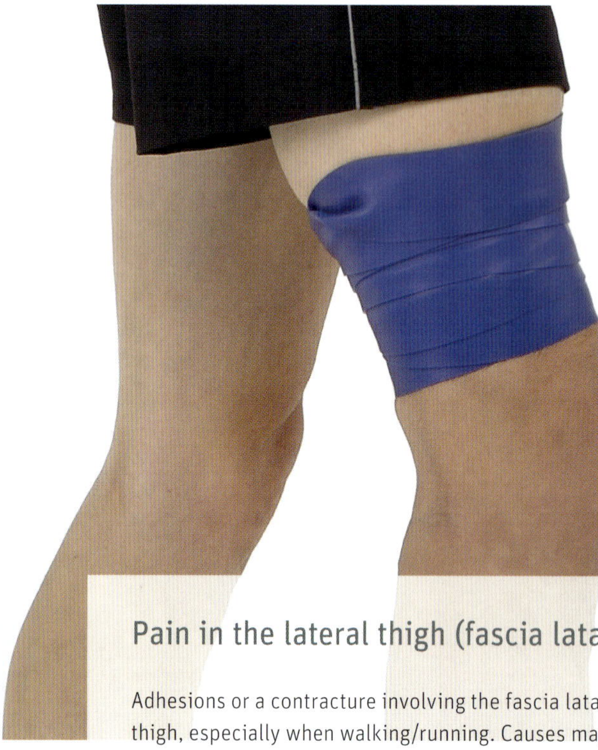

Pain in the lateral thigh (fascia lata)

Adhesions or a contracture involving the fascia lata can lead to pain in the lateral thigh, especially when walking/running. Causes may include inactivity or prolonged abduction of the hip (sitting down).

The flossing band wrap → Here's how it works

1 The patient stands with legs slightly apart. Wind the first turn with 50% tension to anchor the band around the lower part of the thigh.

2 Now wind the flossing band in ascending circular turns. The band should overlap 50% at each turn. Wind the band around the outer thigh with a tension of 60–80%, and with a tension of 50% on the inner side of the thigh.

3 Using the same technique, wind the band further upwards and secure it into place.

Where it hurts on movement

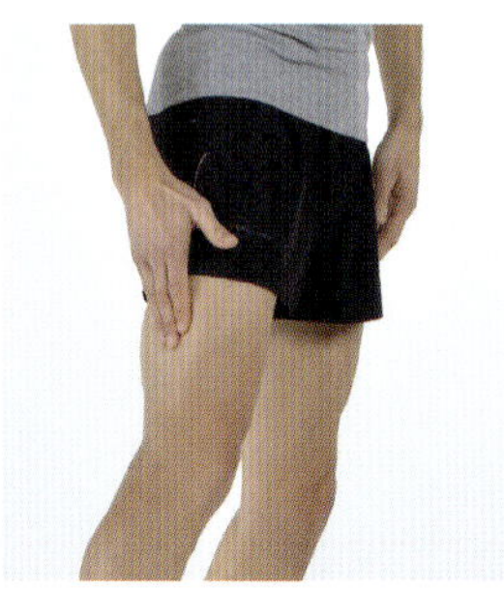

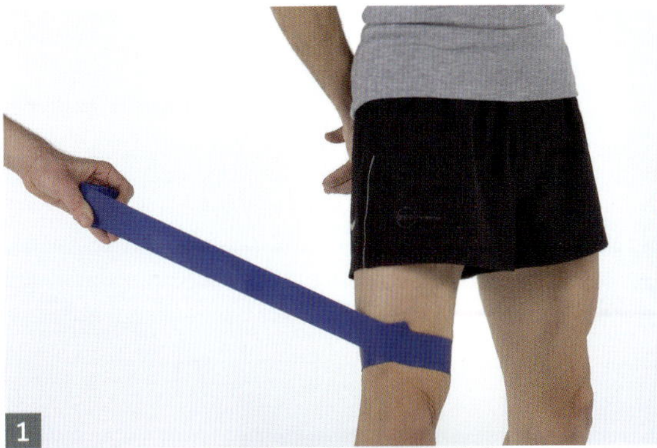
1

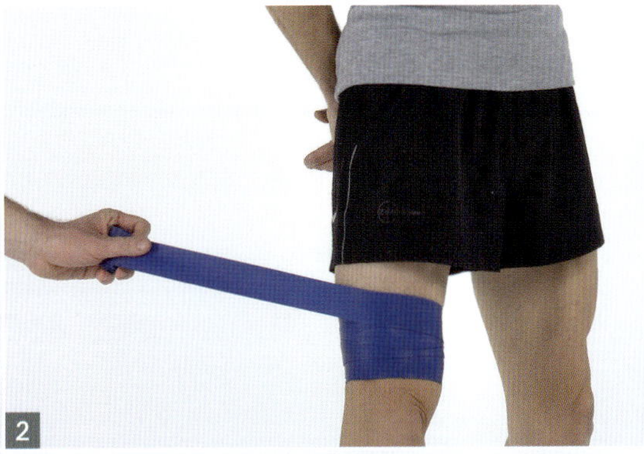
2

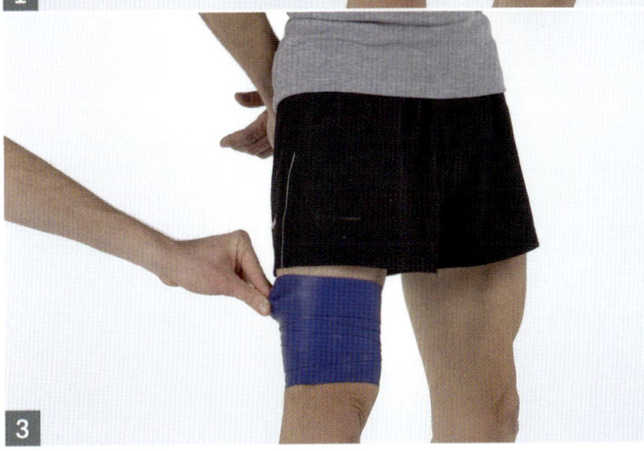
3

Material: Flossing band
Length: 2.06 m
Width: 5 cm
Tension: outside 60–80%, inside 50%

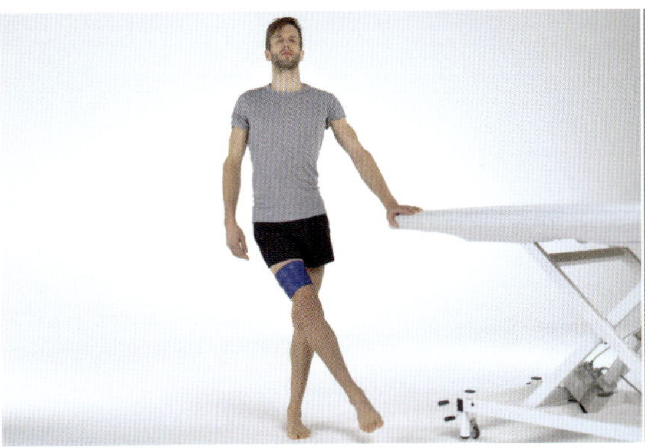

Active Exercise

Move the leg inwards as far as possible and then move it back again. The exercise can be made more dynamic by doing jumping jacks. But you can also walk sideways, crossing one leg over at the front or at the back.

A Word of Advice > When the band is removed, the patient **must** lie down, as the rush of blood into the leg may cause dizziness!

Posterior and anterior thigh muscles

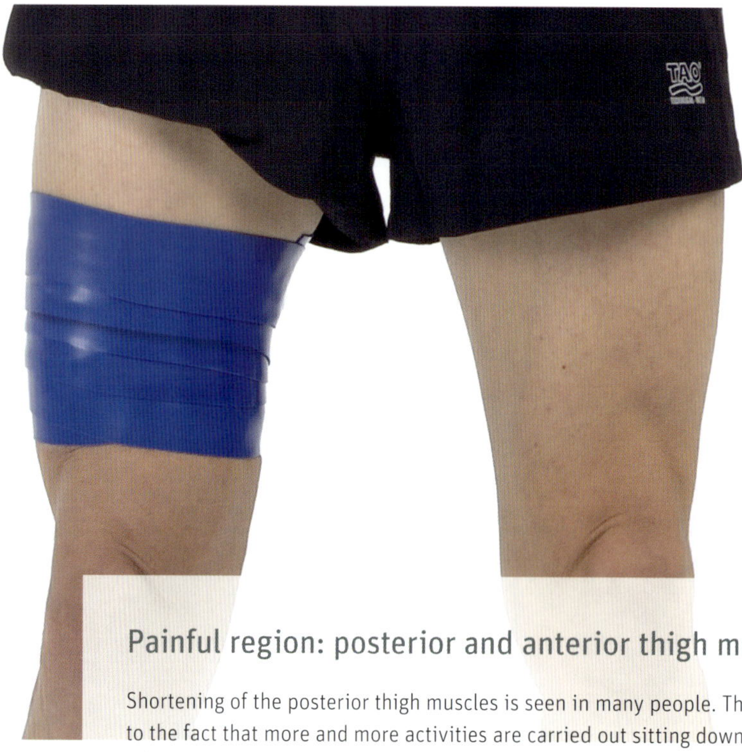

Painful region: posterior and anterior thigh muscles

Shortening of the posterior thigh muscles is seen in many people. This is often due to the fact that more and more activities are carried out sitting down. If these muscles are put to the test in everyday life or during sport, they are often insufficiently flexible and are easily pulled. The anterior thigh muscle (the quadriceps femoris) flexes the knee powerfully and is therefore highly active during walking, running, jumping, climbing stairs, and generally sports. It can become overstrained during these activities. This muscle is also responsible for guiding the movements of the patella. A weakness in the thigh muscle can therefore lead to pain in the muscle itself and also in the patella (see p. 72).

Where it hurts on movement

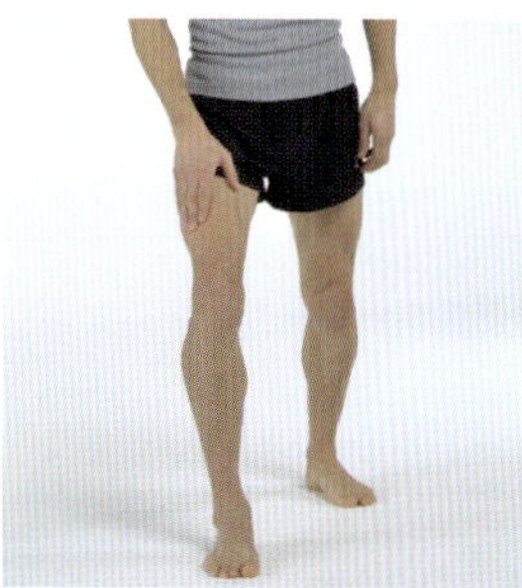

The flossing band wrap ⇢ Here's how it works

1 The patient stands or lies down with legs slightly apart. Wind the first turn with 50% tension to anchor the band around the lower part of the thigh.

2 Now wind the flossing band in circular turns, working up the leg. The band should overlap 50% at each turn. Depending on the site of the pain, wind around the posterior or anterior thigh muscles with a tension of 60.

3 Using the same technique, wind the band further upwards and secure it into place.

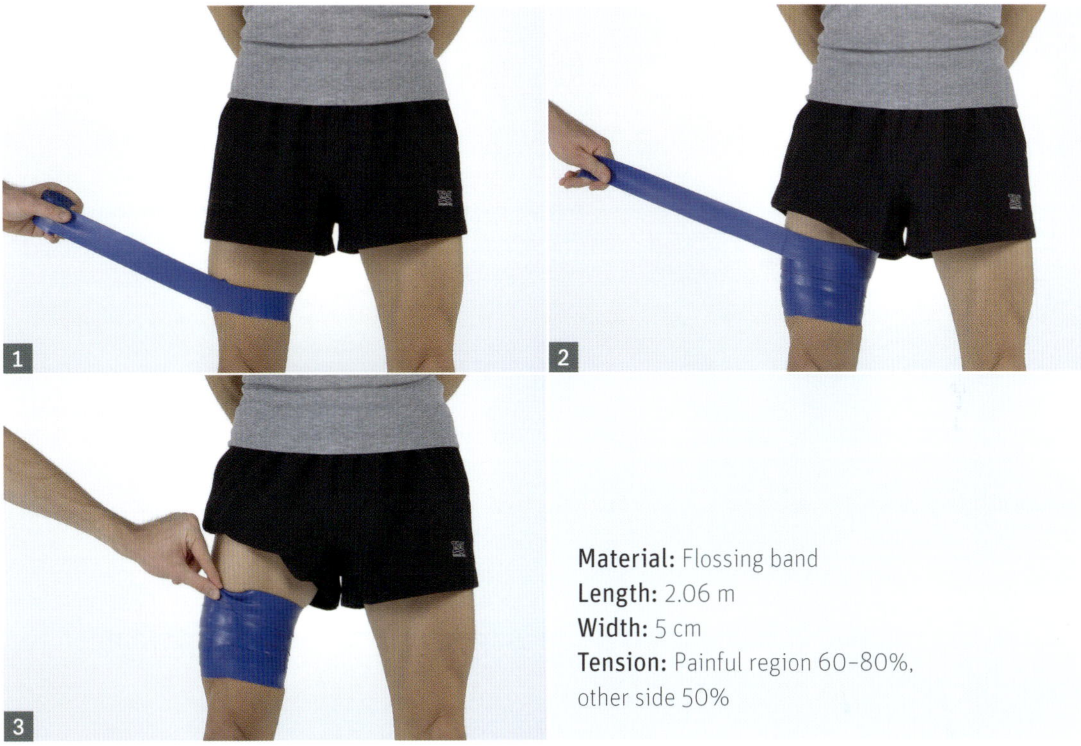

Material: Flossing band
Length: 2.06 m
Width: 5 cm
Tension: Painful region 60–80%, other side 50%

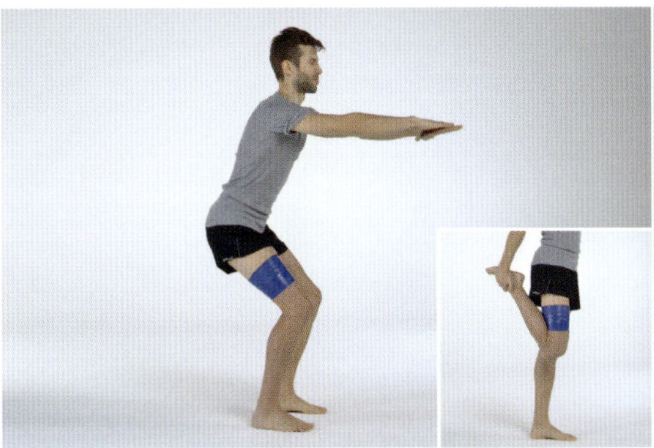

Active Exercise

Do knee bends with both legs at various angles. Alternatively, you can also do single knee bends (lunges). Active stretching exercises are another way of actively moving the knee joint.

A Word of Advice > Weakness of the thigh muscles may lead to knee joint instability and ligament injuries. Therefore, a well-trained muscle is of particular importance in sport.

Knee joint, patella, patellar tendon

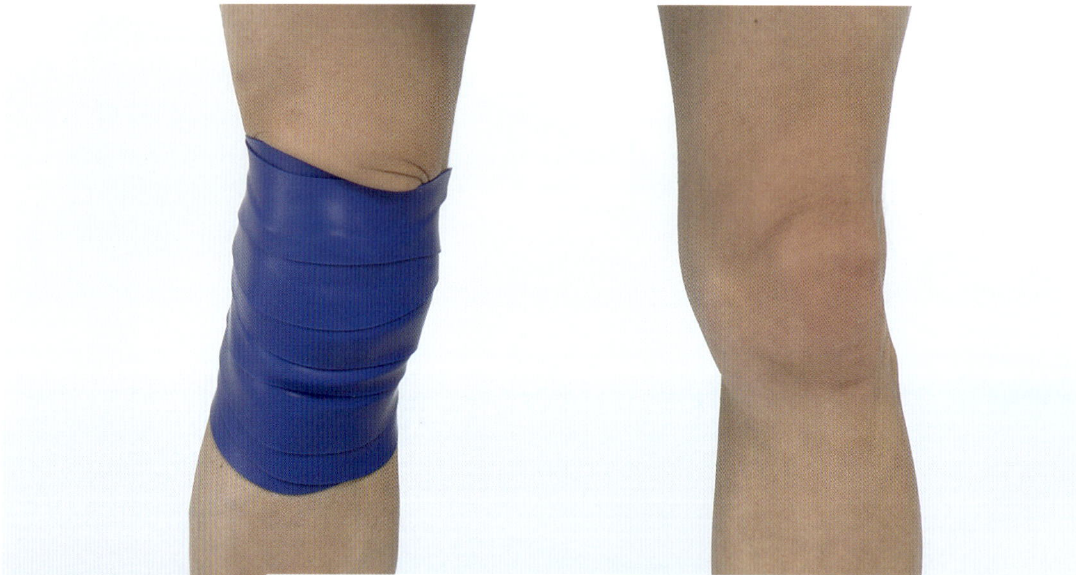

Painful region: knee joint, patella, patellar tendon

Knee pain can have a variety of causes. These are frequently functional, rather than structural causes such as osteoarthritis. If pain is experienced on the lateral side or behind the patella when walking, climbing stairs, or during sport, the reason may be that the patella is not gliding correctly in its groove. Muscular imbalances or irritation of the tendons that surround the patella can cause this pain. Pain in the patellar tendon often results from overload.

The flossing band wrap ⇢ Here's how it works

1 The patient lies supine with the knee extended. Support the leg so that the knee hangs free. Wind the first turn with 50% tension to anchor it below the knee.

2 Now wind the flossing band in ascending circular turns. The band should overlap 50% at each turn. Depending on the site of the pain, wind the band around the patellar tendon or the patella itself with a tension of 60–80%, and with a tension of 50% on the dorsal side of the knee. Using the same technique, wind the band further upwards to enclose the whole knee and secure it into place.

3 If the cause of the knee pain is unknown or if the pain is located slightly above the patella, the wrap may also be applied using the "open technique", i.e. leaving the patella itself unwrapped.

Painful movement

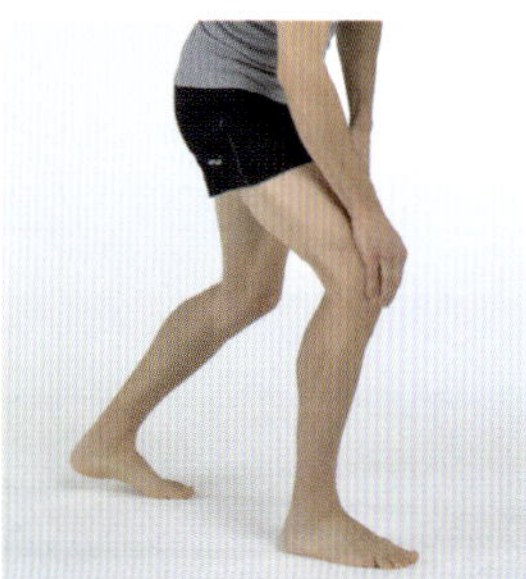

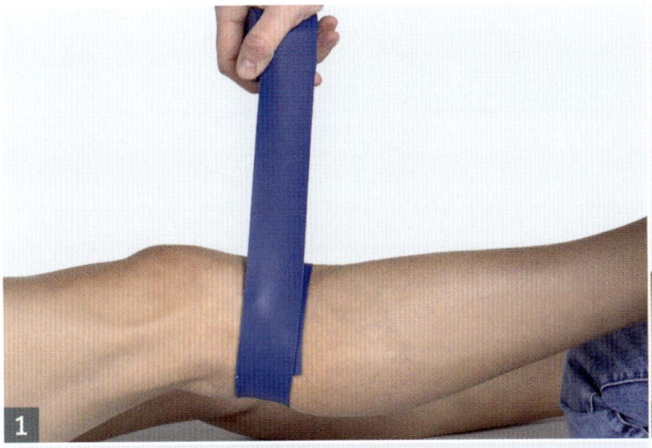

1

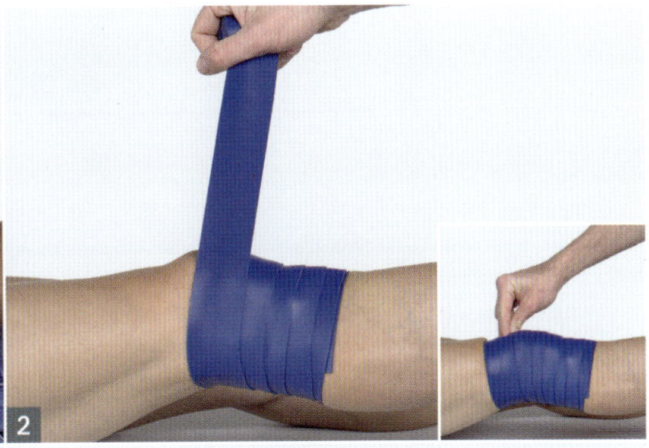

2

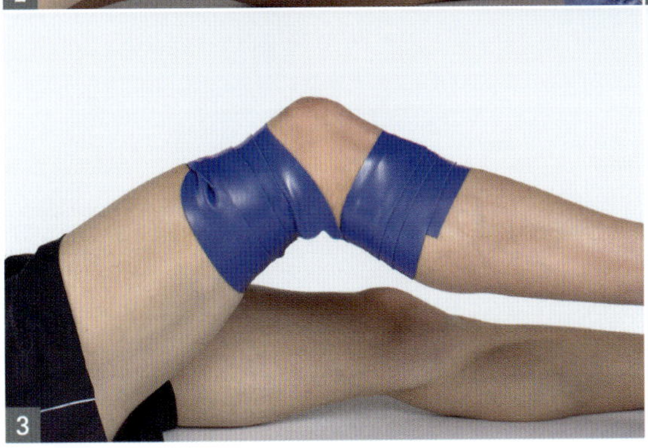

3

Material: Flossing band
Length: 2.06 m
Width: 5 cm
Tension: Front 60–80%, back 50%

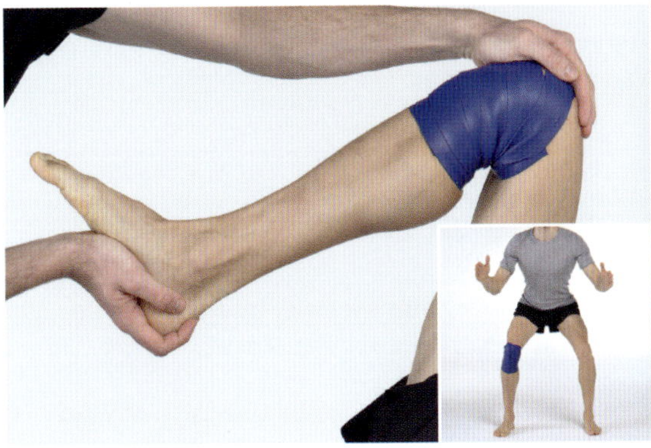

Active Exercise

As an active exercise, you can do gentle frog jumps or try out a variety of knee bends. You can also walk on uneven ground or take big forward steps.

A Word of Advice > If only the patellar tendon hurts, the wrap may be restricted to this region alone.

Medial collateral ligament of the knee, medial meniscus

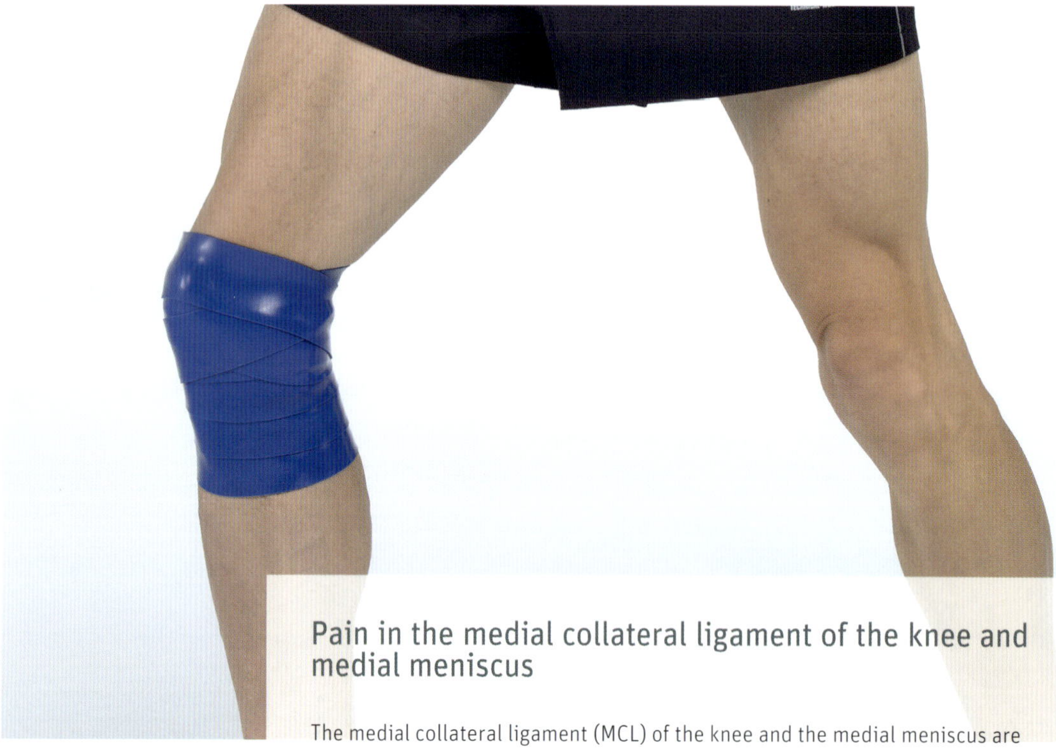

Pain in the medial collateral ligament of the knee and medial meniscus

The medial collateral ligament (MCL) of the knee and the medial meniscus are easily injured if a sideways force acts on the knee. This can happen in contacts sports such as martial arts, but also in ball games. A varus deformity of the knee (or sitting cross-legged) stresses the medial meniscus, while knock knees mean an increased strain on the MCL.

The flossing band wrap → Here's how it works

1 The patient lies supine with the knee extended. Support the leg so that the knee hangs free. Wind the first turn with 50% tension to anchor it around the top of the lower leg.

2 Now wind the flossing band in circular turns, working up the leg. The band should overlap 50% at each turn. Wind the band with a tension of 60–80% on the inner (medial) side of the knee, and with a tension of 50% on the dorsal and outer (lateral) sides of the knee.

3 Using the same technique, wind the band further upwards to enclose the whole knee and secure it into place.

Where it hurts on movement

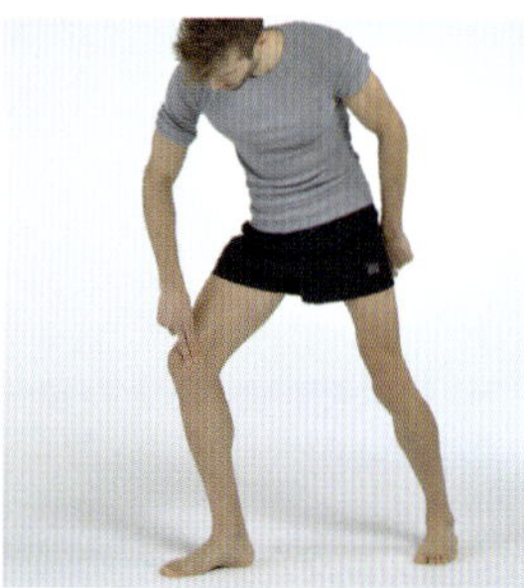

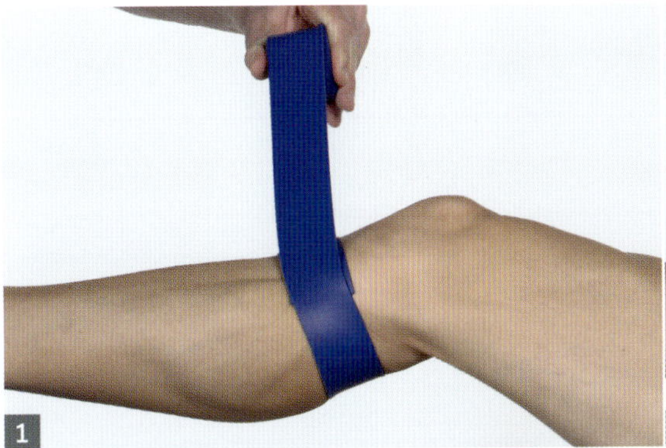

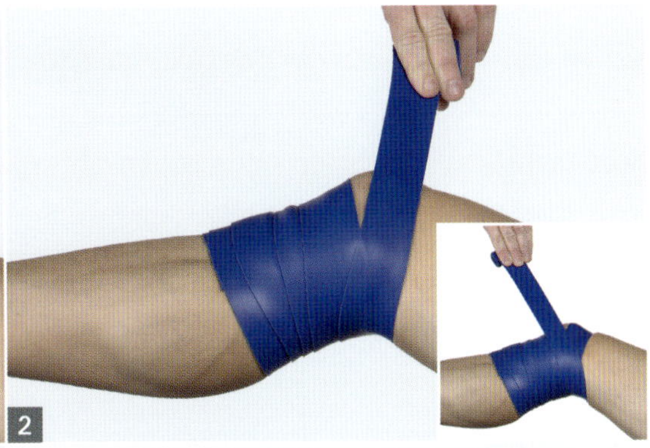

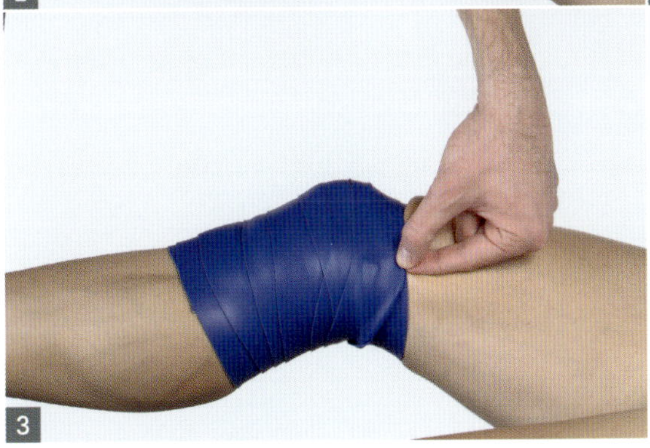

Material: Flossing band
Length: 2.06 m
Width: 5 cm
Tension: Inside 60–80%, outside 50%

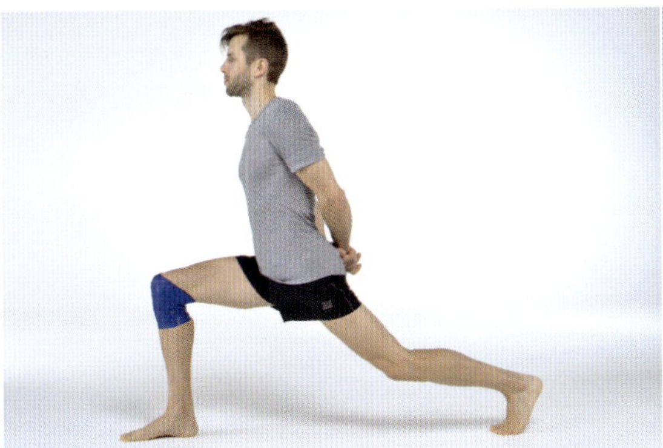

Active Exercise

Take a big forward step and do deep knee bends (lunges).

A Word of Advice > The flossing band may also be crossed over several times on the inner (medial) side of the knee (step 2, small image).

Lateral collateral ligament of the knee, lateral meniscus

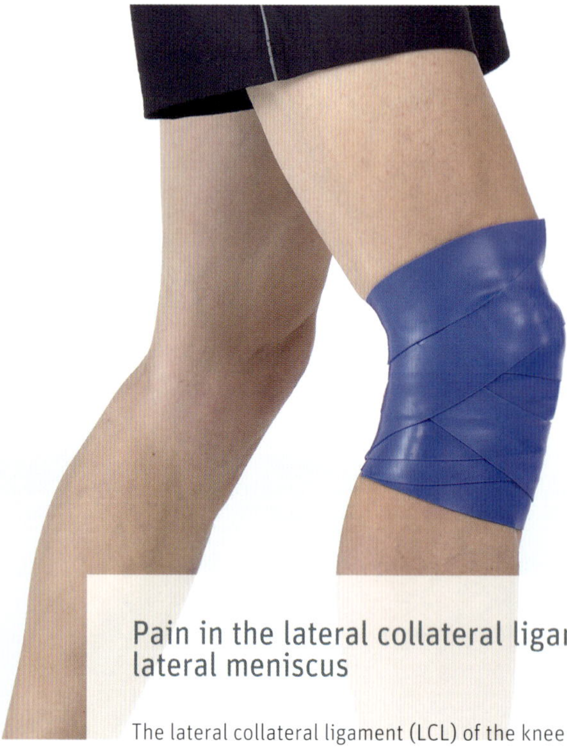

Pain in the lateral collateral ligament of the knee and lateral meniscus

The lateral collateral ligament (LCL) of the knee and the lateral meniscus are easily injured if a sideways force acts on the knee. This can happen in contacts sports such as martial arts, but also in ball games. A valgus deformity of the knee stresses the lateral meniscus, while bow legs or sitting cross-legged mean an increased strain on the LCL.

The flossing band wrap ⇢ Here's how it works

1 The patient lies supine with the knee extended. Support the leg so that the knee hangs free. Wind the first turn with 50% tension to anchor it around the top of the lower leg.

Where it hurts on movement

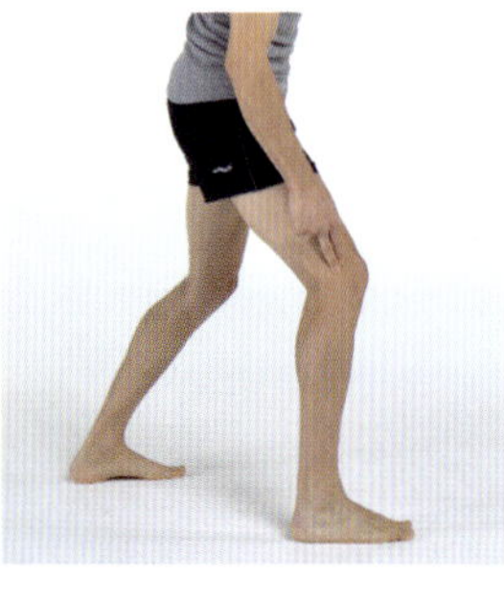

2 Now wind the flossing band in ascending circular turns. The band should overlap 50% at each turn. Wind the band with a tension of 60–80% on the outer (lateral) side of the knee, and with a tension of 50% on the posterior and inner (medial) sides of the knee.

3 Using the same technique, wind the band further upwards to enclose the whole knee and secure it into place.

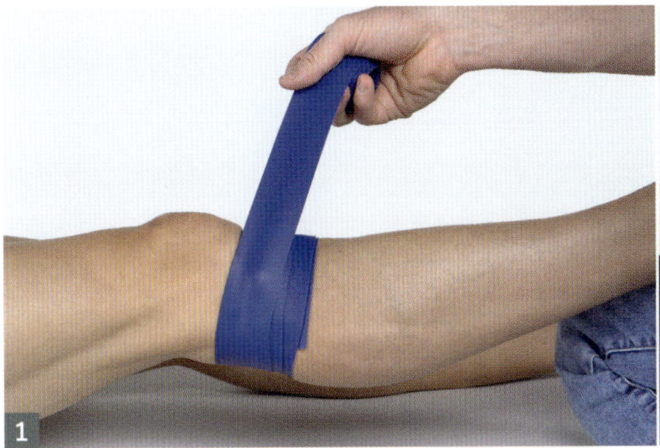

1

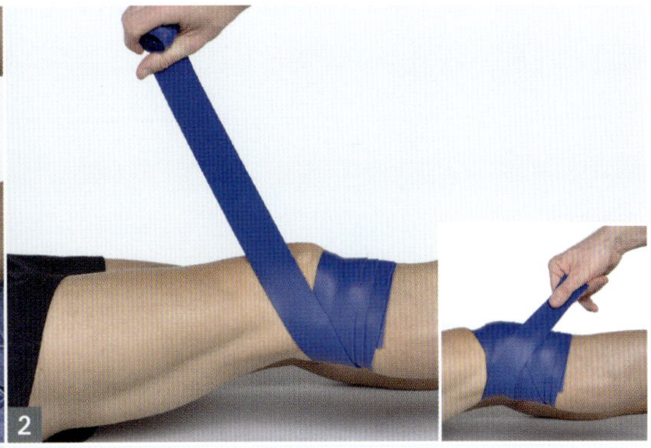

2

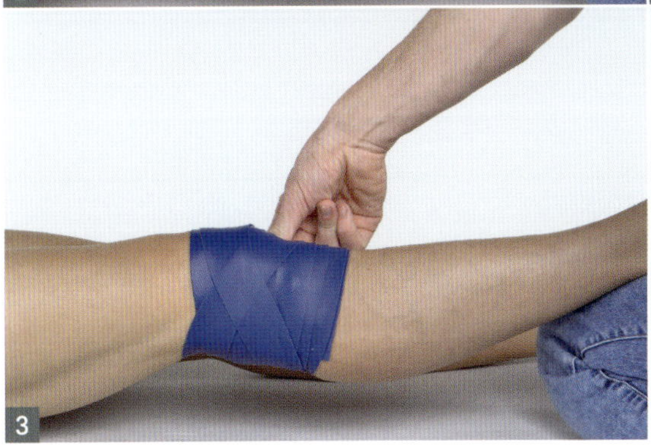

3

Material: Flossing band
Length: 2.06 m
Width: 5 cm
Tension: Outside 60–80%, inside 50%

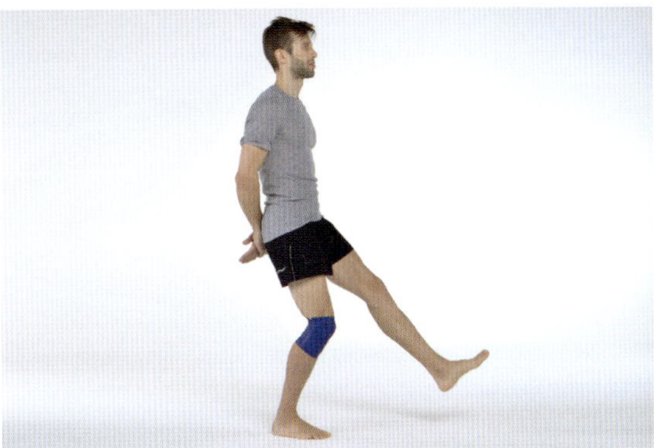

Active Exercise

Stand on the flossed leg, stabilize the knee, and perform a deep knee bend.

A Word of Advice > The flossing band may also be crossed over several times on the outer (lateral) side of the knee (step 2, small image).

Calf muscles

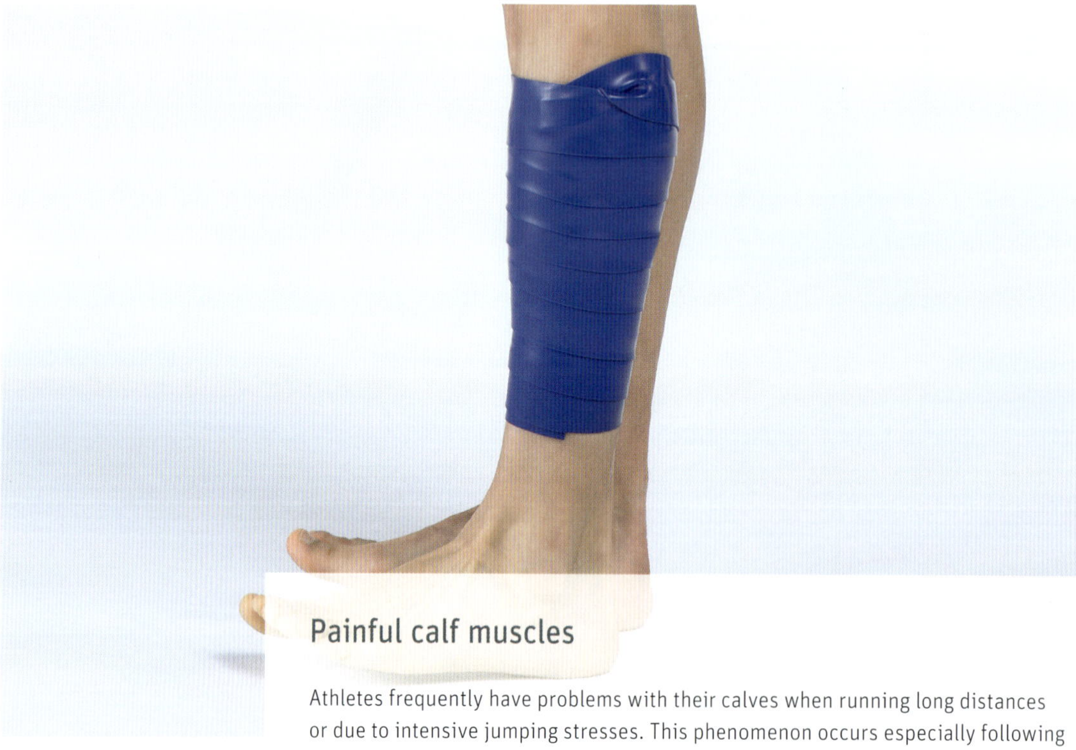

Painful calf muscles

Athletes frequently have problems with their calves when running long distances or due to intensive jumping stresses. This phenomenon occurs especially following long pauses in training. The regular "pushing off" with the feet can lead to excess strain in the calf muscles, particularly during hill running. Since the power of the calf muscles is transferred to the foot predominantly by the Achilles tendon, the latter can also become painful.

The flossing band wrap → Here's how it works

1 The patient lies supine, the knee is slightly flexed and the foot is on the couch. Wind the first turn with 50% tension to anchor it around the bottom part of the lower leg.

Painful movement

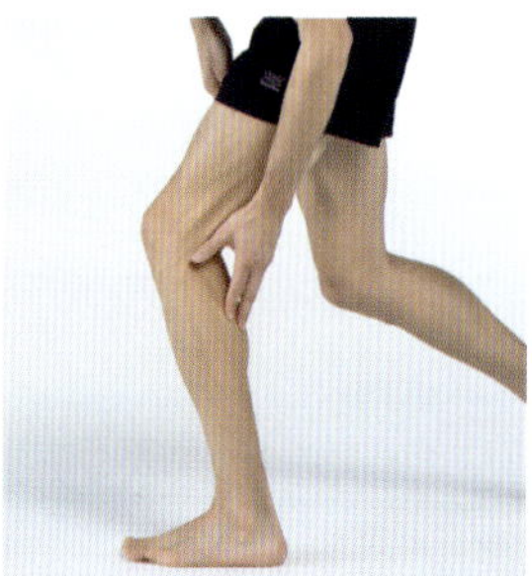

2 Now wind the flossing band in ascending circular turns. The band should overlap 50% at each turn. Wind the band with a tension of 60–80% on the posterior side of the lower leg, and with a tension of 50% on the anterior side.

3 Using the same technique, wind the band further upwards to enclose the calf muscles in full and secure it into place.

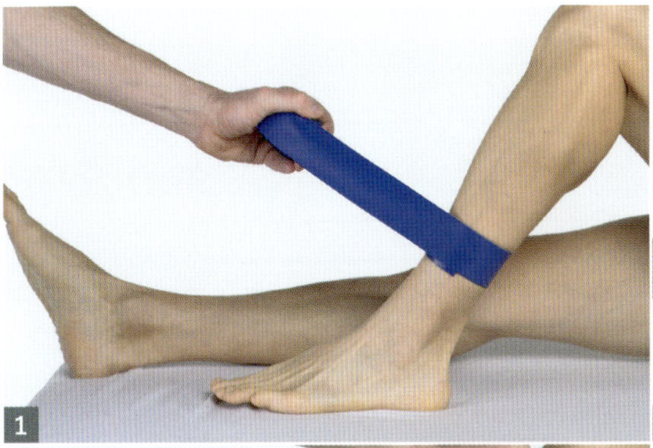
1

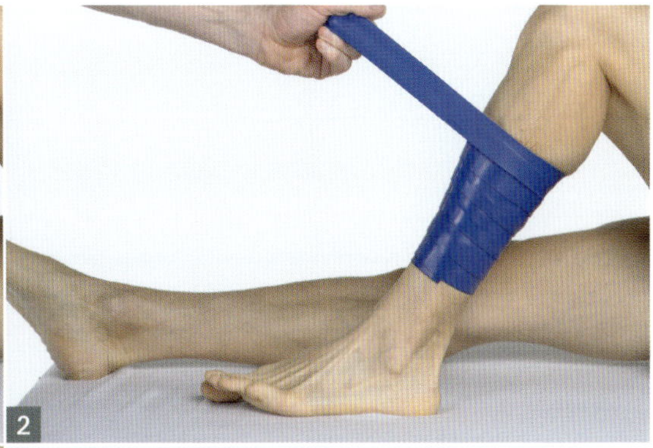
2

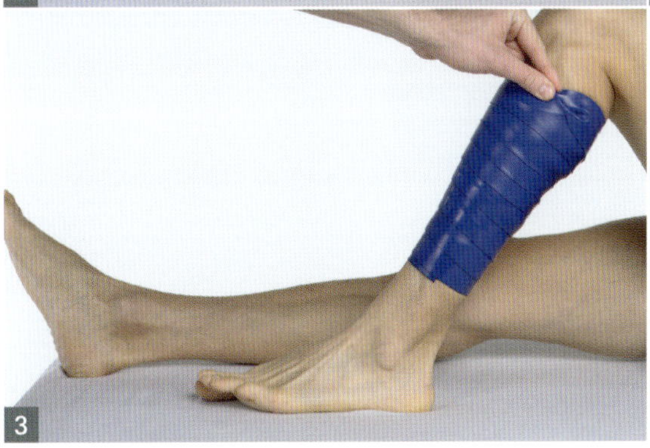
3

Material: Flossing band
Length: 2.06 m
Width: 5 cm
Tension: Back 60–80%, front 50%

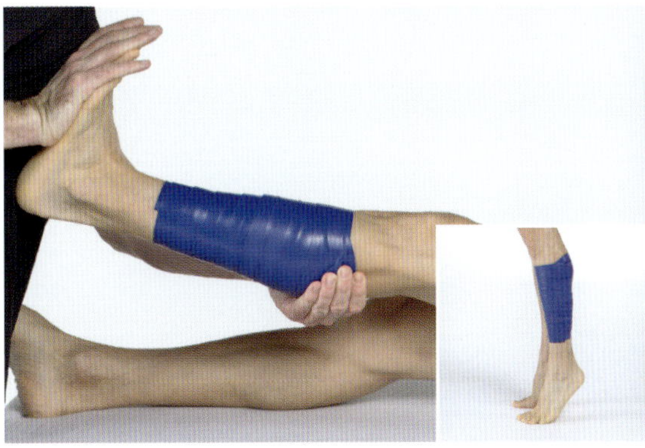

Active Exercise

Walk alternately on your toes and heels. Do several active toe stands. You can also perform active stretches in flexion and extension.

A Word of Advice > Wearing high-heeled shoes encourages shortening of the calf muscles and should be avoided.

Achilles tendon

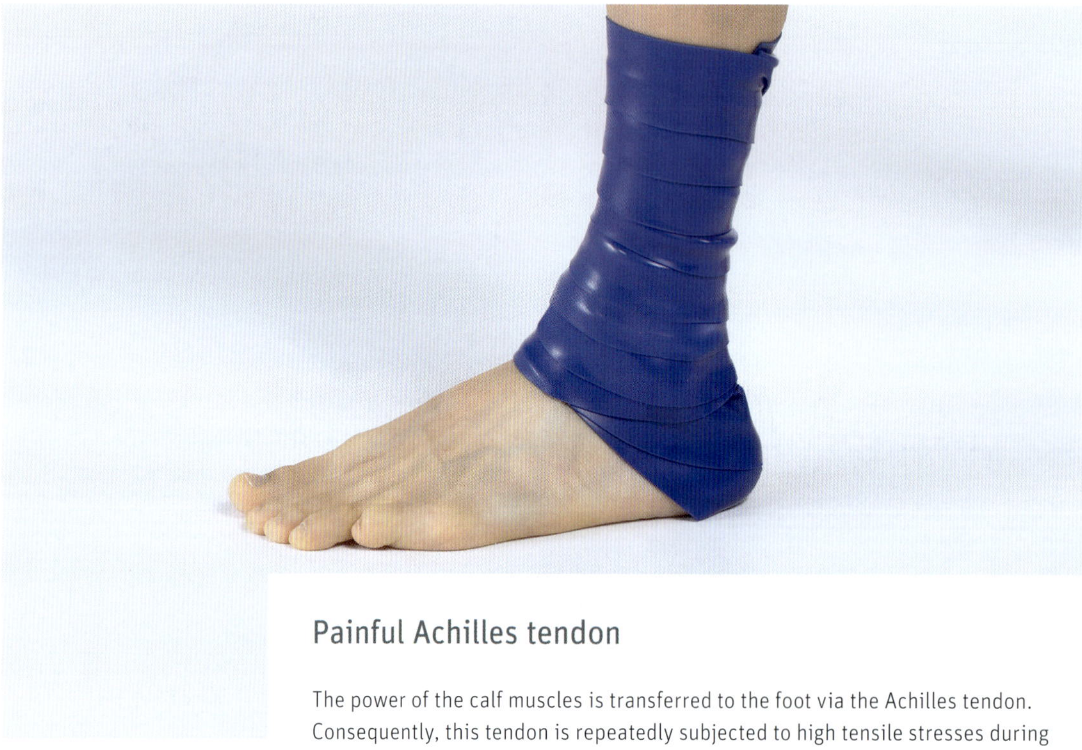

Painful Achilles tendon

The power of the calf muscles is transferred to the foot via the Achilles tendon. Consequently, this tendon is repeatedly subjected to high tensile stresses during running and jumping. Athletes (particularly sprinters) who run predominantly on the forefoot subject the tendon to particularly high strains. The pain may be located in the tendon itself and also at its junction with the heel bone (calcaneus).

The flossing band wrap ⇢ Here's how it works

1 The patient lies supine or prone, the foot hangs over the edge of the therapy couch. The patient should pull the foot up slightly. Wind the first turn with 50% tension to anchor it around the ankle and the heel bone.

2 Now wind the flossing band in ascending circular turns. The band should overlap 50% at each turn. Wind the band with a tension of 60–80% in the region of the Achilles tendon and the back of the lower leg, and with a tension of 50% on its anterior side.

3 Using the same technique, continue winding the band up to the middle of the lower leg and secure it into place there.

Painful movement

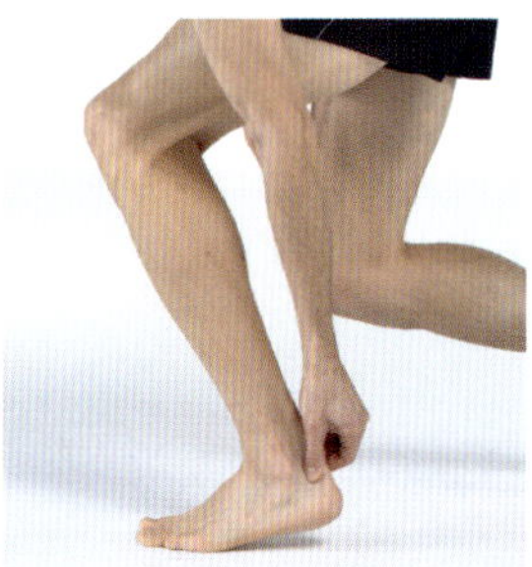

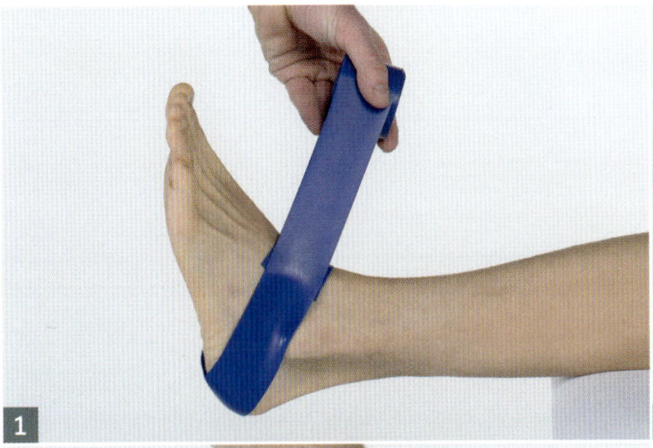
1

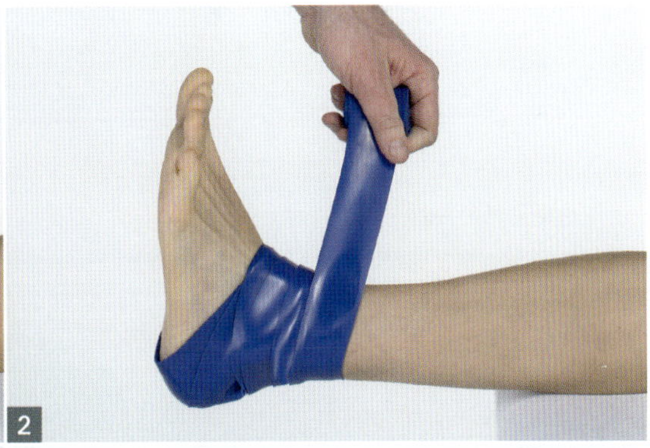
2

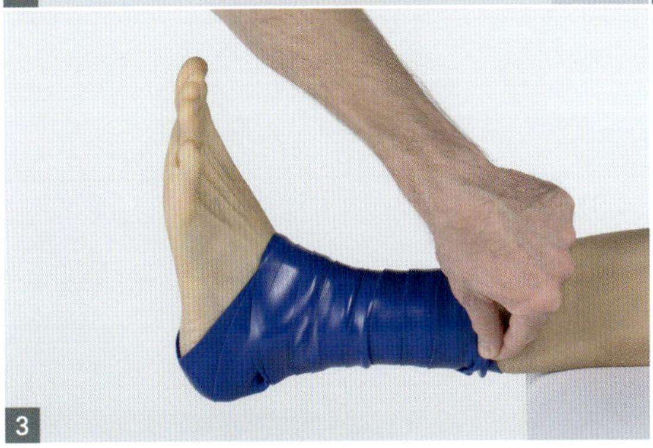
3

Material: Flossing band
Length: 2.06 m
Width: 5 cm
Tension: Back 60–80%, front 50%

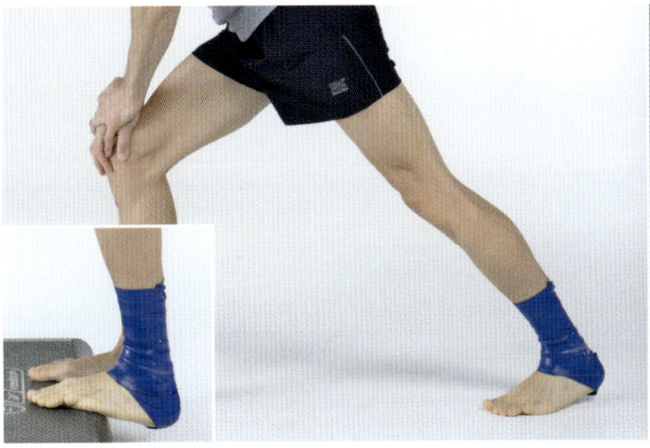

Active Exercise

Take a big step backwards (lunge), put your foot down and stretch your calf muscles and Achilles tendon; alternatively, stretch the tendon on a stair tread or stepper machine, by pushing the heels down as far as possible (small image). You can also bring yourself into a toe stand and then slowly let the feet sink to the floor (eccentric training).

A Word of Advice > You could also perform the calf muscle exercises. If the main site of the pain is directly on the heel bone, you may have bursitis. If this is the case, consult a doctor.

Ankle joint

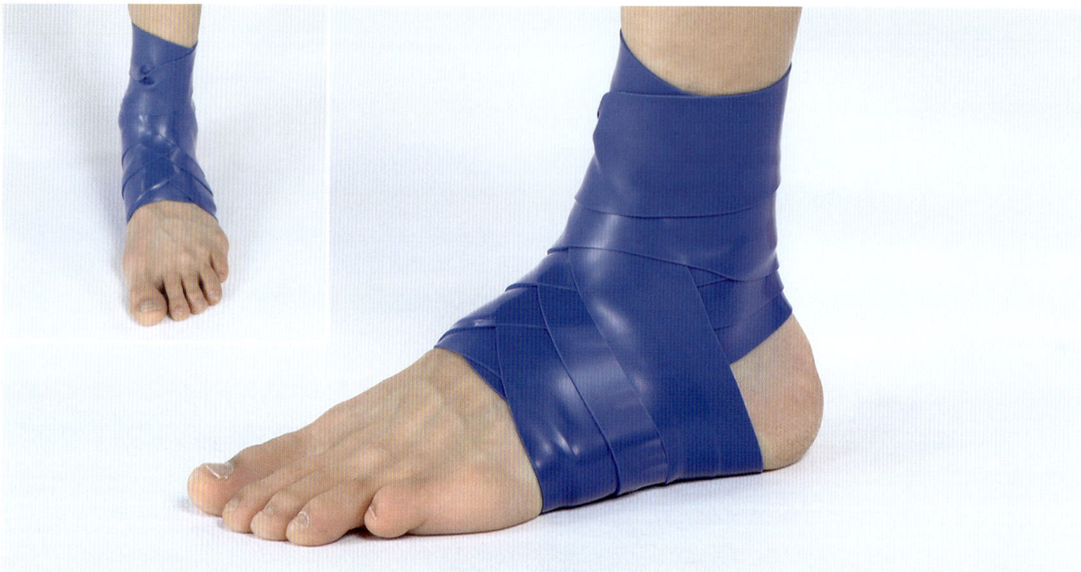

Painful region: ankle joint

Pain in the ankle joint region frequently develops following ligament injuries (see p. 84). Injuries to the ligaments and the joint capsule, or ankle joint fractures (Weber B, Maisonneuve etc.) which have not healed properly, can cause pain on weight-bearing. Flossing can accelerate the healing process, but should only be used alongside other treatment measures.

The flossing band wrap → Here's how it works

1 The patient lies supine, the foot hangs over the edge of the therapy couch. The patient should pull the foot up slightly. Wind the first turn with 50% tension to anchor it around the metatarsus.

2 Now wind the flossing band in figure-of-eight turns around the lower leg and back again to the foot. The band should overlap 50% at each turn. Wind the band with a tension of 60–80% where the pain is most intense and with a tension of 50% on the other side.

3 Using the same technique, continue winding the band to the end and secure it into place.

Where it hurts on weight-bearing

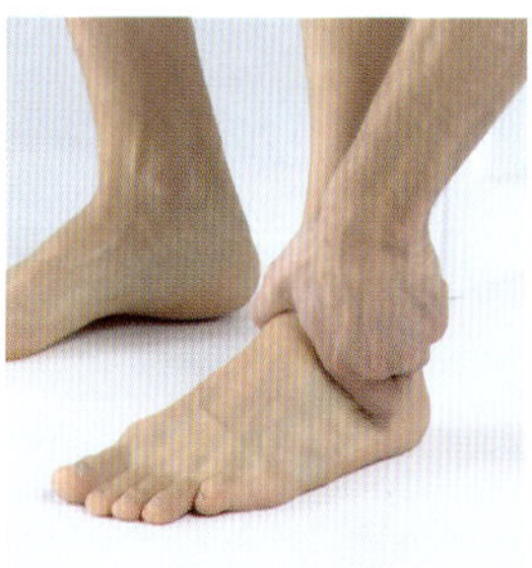

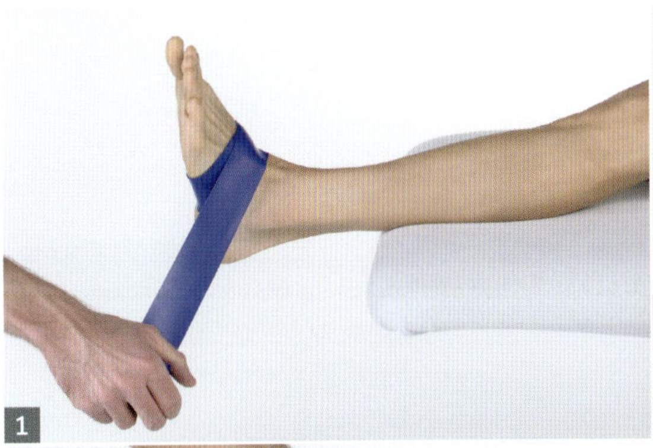
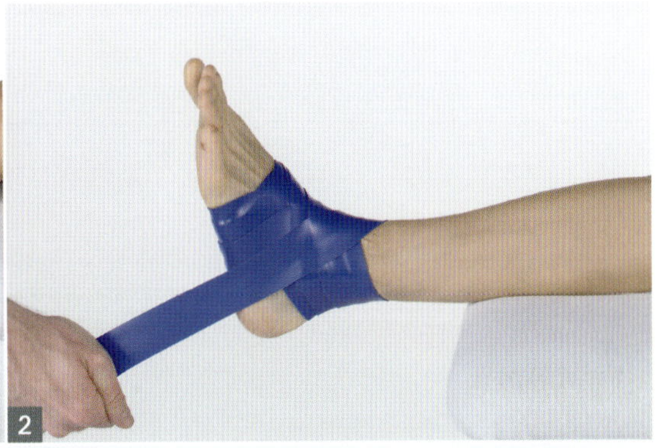
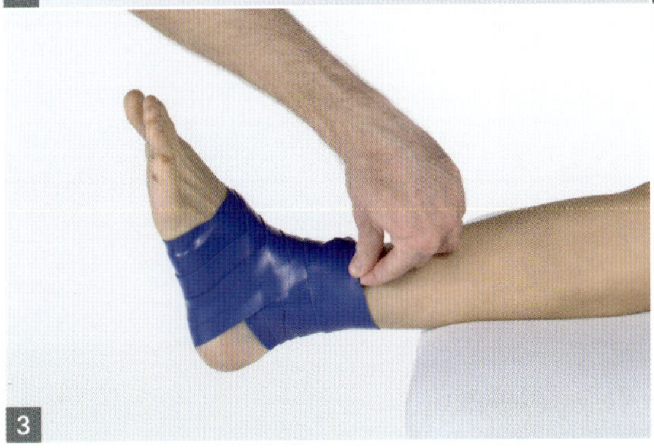

Material: Flossing band
Length: 2.06 m
Width: 5 cm
Tension: Painful region 60–80%, other side 50%

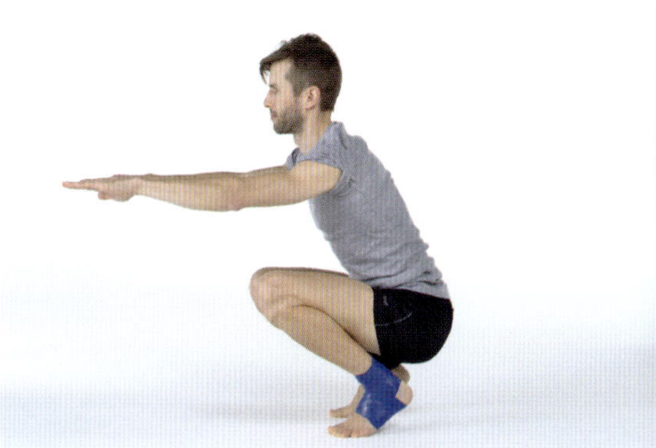

Active Exercise

Do deep knee bends or duck walking. An alternative option is to perform alternate toe and heel stands. In addition, you can make circles with your feet while sitting or lying down.

A Word of Advice > Wrapping the forefoot too tightly can lead to compression pain, so that the wrap should be a bit looser in this region.

Twisted ankle (supination/pronation trauma)

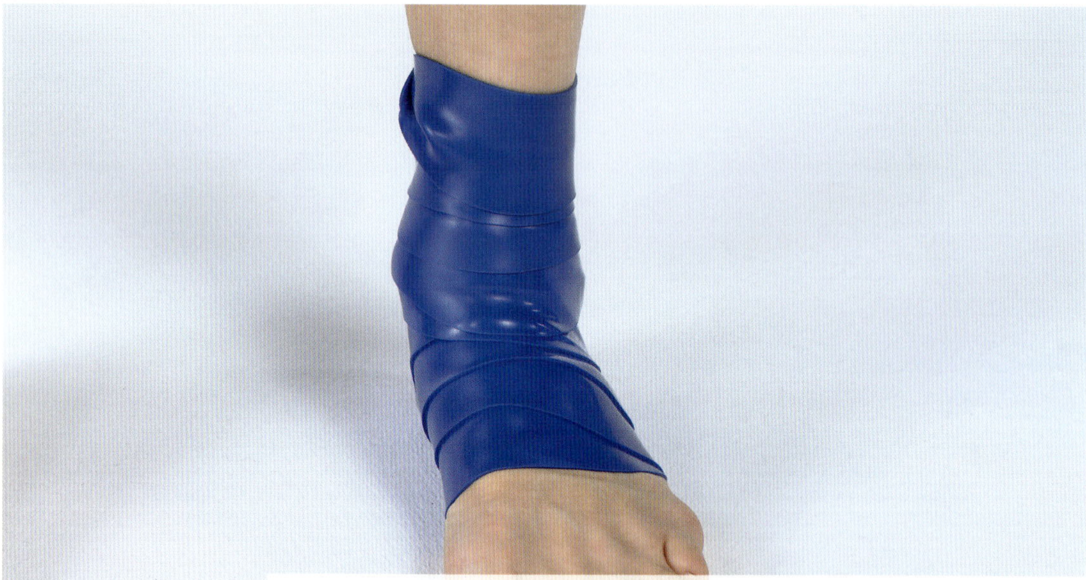

Twisted ankle (supination/pronation trauma)

Pain in the ankle joint is often the result of a twisted ankle, which causes overstretching of the lateral capsule and ligamentous structures of the ankle joint. This is known as supination trauma, i.e. twisting the ankle outwards. Twisting in the opposite direction (pronation trauma) is less common. A twisted ankle can be caused by muscular imbalances in the lower leg and foot muscles. Twisting of the ankle should be taken seriously, as the ligaments and joint capsule are repeatedly injured and the ankle becomes more and more unstable with time or with each new twisting injury.

The flossing band wrap ⇢ Here's how it works

1 The patient lies supine, the foot hangs over the edge of the therapy couch. The patient should pull the foot up slightly. Wind the first turn with 50% tension to anchor it around the forefoot. Important: in supination trauma, the band should be wound so that the foot is pulled into pronation.

2 Now wind the flossing band in ascending circular turns. The band should overlap 50% at each turn. In supination trauma, wind the band with a tension of 60–80% over the

3 Using the same technique, wind the band up to the lower leg and secure it into place there.

Where it hurts on movement

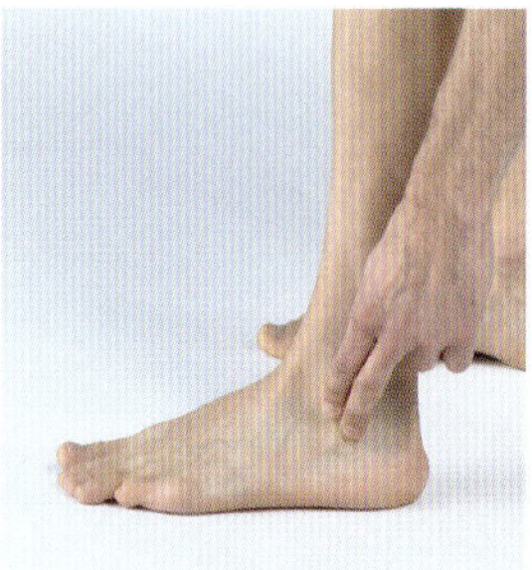

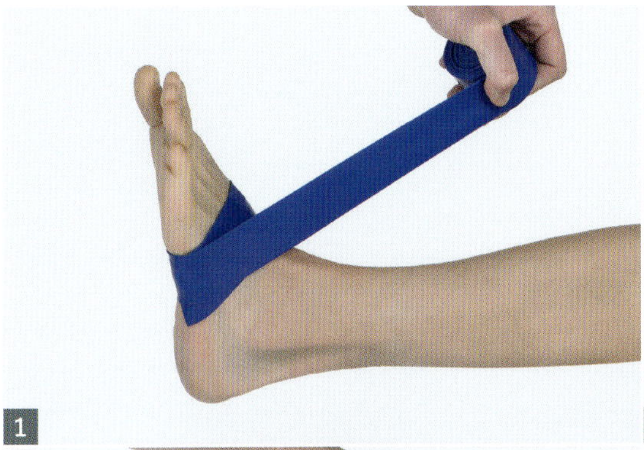

1

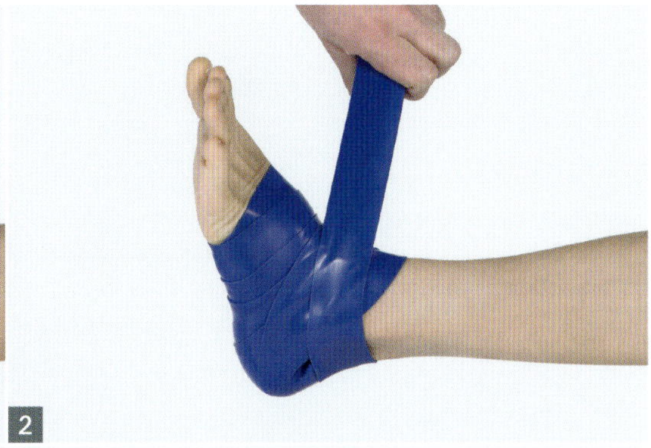

2

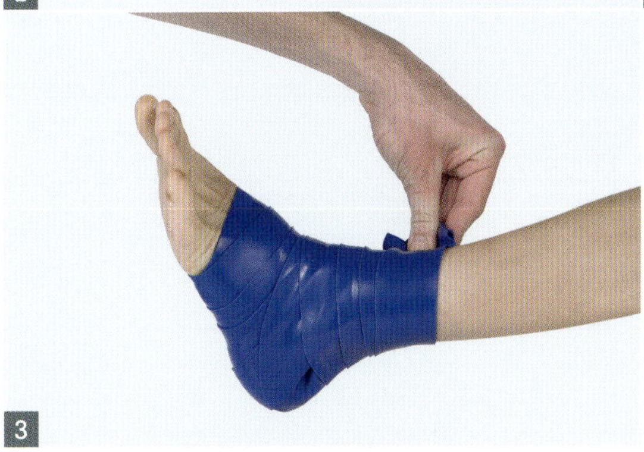

3

Material: Flossing band
Length: 2.06 m
Width: 5 cm
Tension: Painful region 60–80%, other side 50%

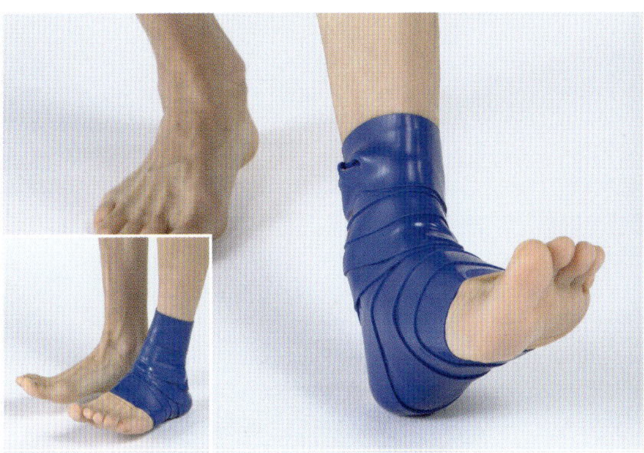

Active Exercise

Make circling movements with the foot while sitting or lying down. You can also walk on the inner or outer side of the foot on a soft surface.

A Word of Advice > In pronation trauma, wind the band around the foot the other way (pulling the foot into supination); the main pull of the band should then be over the medial malleolus.

Heel spur, plantar aponeurosis

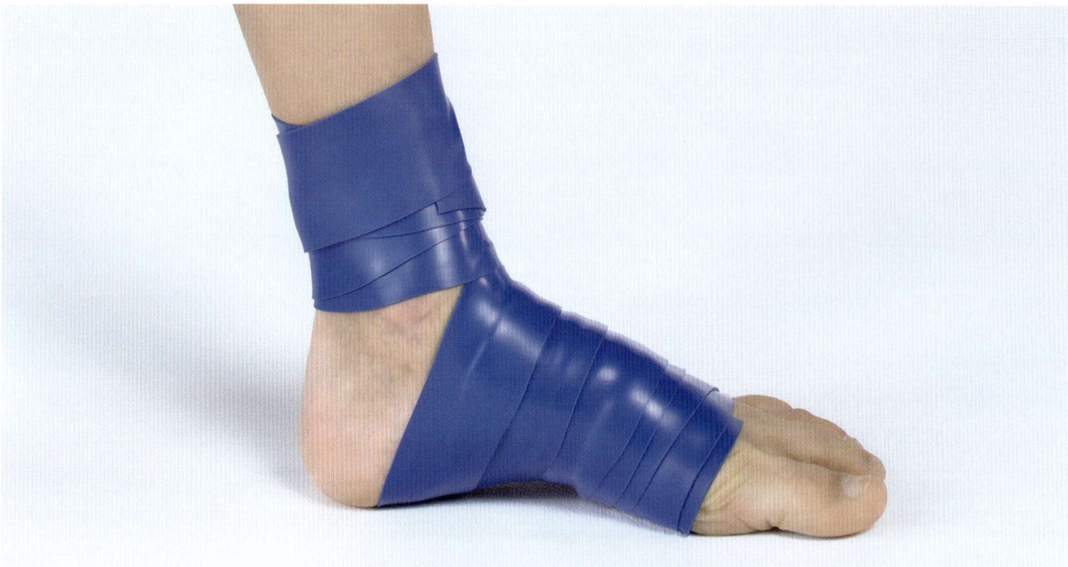

Heel spur, plantar aponeurosis

Muscular imbalances, lack of exercise, or being overweight are just a few examples of factors that can lead to flattening of the longitudinal and transverse arches of the feet. Fallen arches then cause stretching of the ligaments on the underside of the foot, e.g. the plantar aponeurosis. This is generally associated with severe pain in the heel bone, where a heel spur frequently forms at the bone's junction with the plantar aponeurosis, as a result of the high tensile stress involved.

The flossing band wrap ⇢ Here's how it works

1 The patient lies supine, the foot hangs over the edge of the therapy couch. The patient should pull the foot up slightly. Wind the first turn with 50% tension to anchor it around the forefoot.

2 Now wind the flossing band in ascending circular turns. The band should overlap 50% at each turn. Wind the band with a tension of 60–80% over the sole of the foot, and with a tension of 50% over the dorsum of the foot.

3 Using the same technique, wind the band over the ankle and up to the lower leg and secure it into place there.

Where it hurts
on weight-bearing

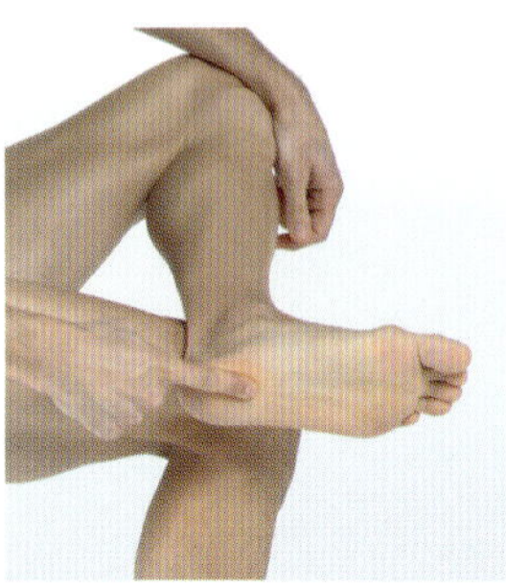

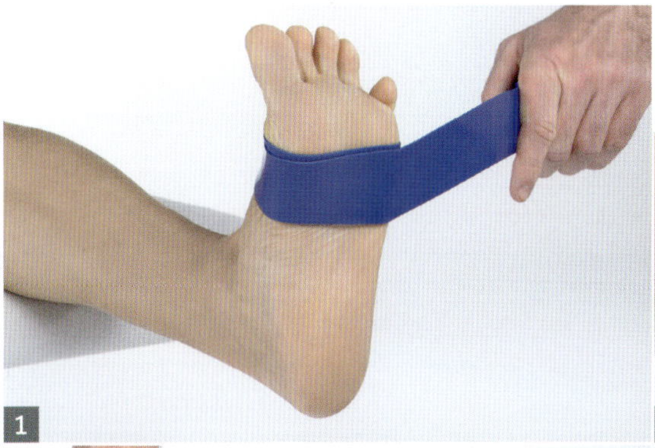

1

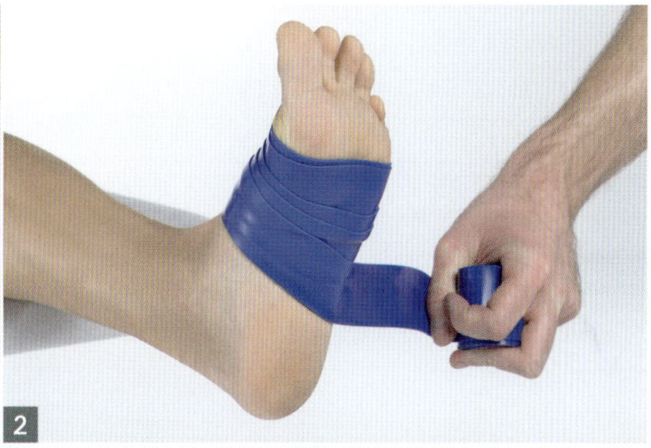

2

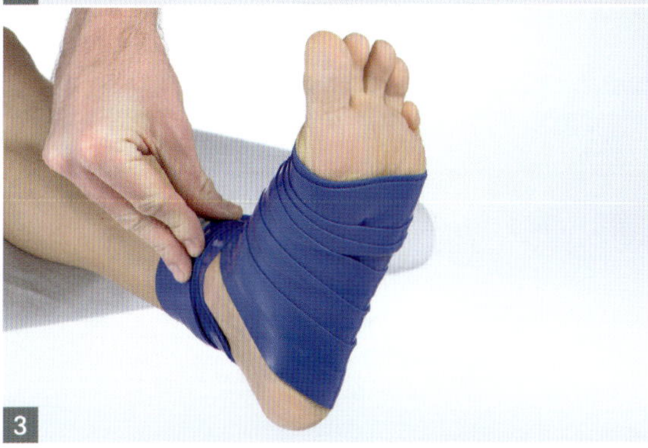

3

Material: Flossing band
Length: 2.06 m
Width: 5 cm
Tension: Sole of the foot 60–80%, other side 50%

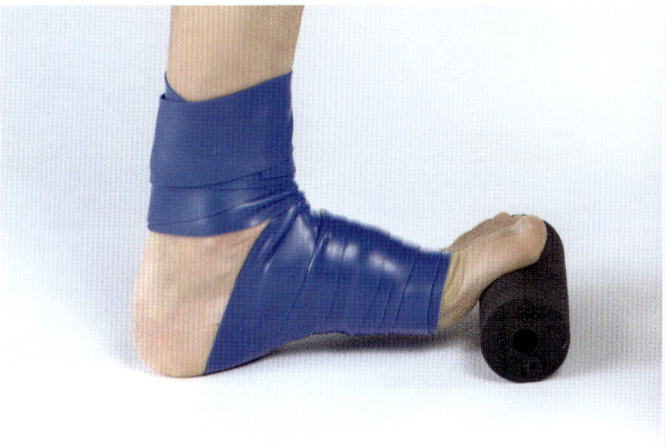

Active Exercise

Stretch the calf and foot muscles by stepping back slightly, putting the foot down and placing the forefoot and toes on a roller. In addition, you can also roll out the sole of the foot with a fascia roller or tennis ball. The pain experienced while doing so should still be just about bearable. Active stretches are an added alternative here.

A Word of Advice > Insoles can correct the shape of the foot mechanically and give it support. However, it is very important to activate the foot muscles to achieve a good long-term result.

Hallux valgus (bunion), toe joints

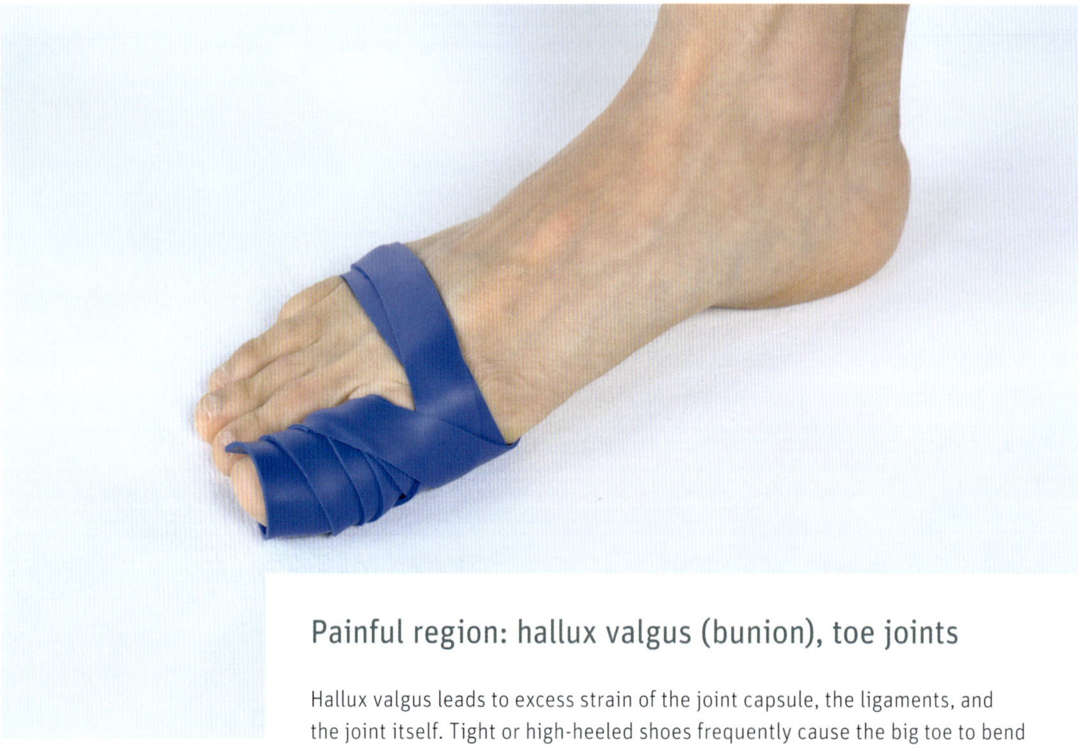

Painful region: hallux valgus (bunion), toe joints

Hallux valgus leads to excess strain of the joint capsule, the ligaments, and the joint itself. Tight or high-heeled shoes frequently cause the big toe to bend inwards, but fallen arches (splayfoot or talipes valgus) can also produce this situation. A familial predisposition is common, in which case it is even more important to start self-treating at an early stage

The flossing band wrap → Here's how it works

1 The patient lies supine, the leg lies on the therapy couch. Wind the first turn with 50% tension to anchor the band around the big toe.

2 Now wind the flossing band further around the toe in a second circular turn. The band should overlap 50%. Take the third turn around the anterior forefoot, then another turn around the toe. Wind the band around the toe joints on the medial side of the foot with a tension of 60–80%; otherwise, apply a tension of 50%.

3 Using the same technique, wind the band further around the forefoot up the end and secure it into place there.

Where it hurts
on weight-bearing

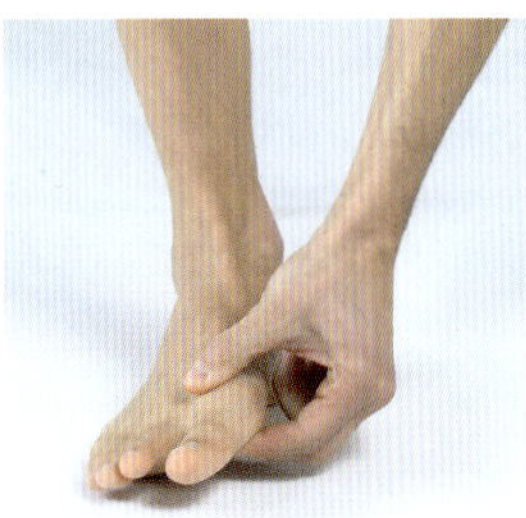

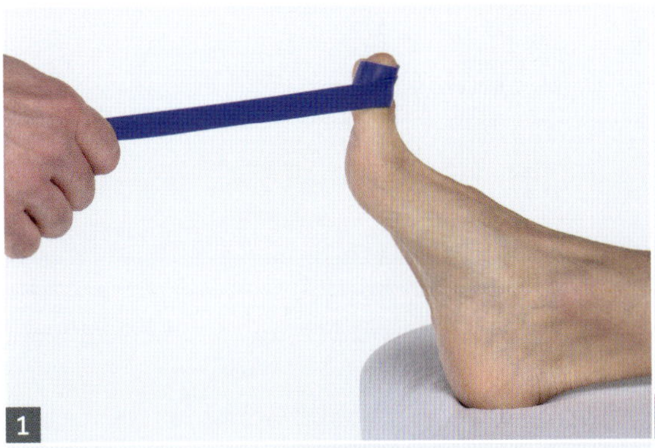

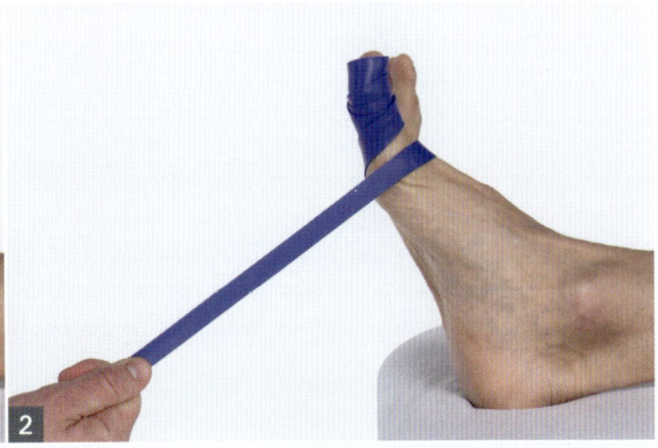

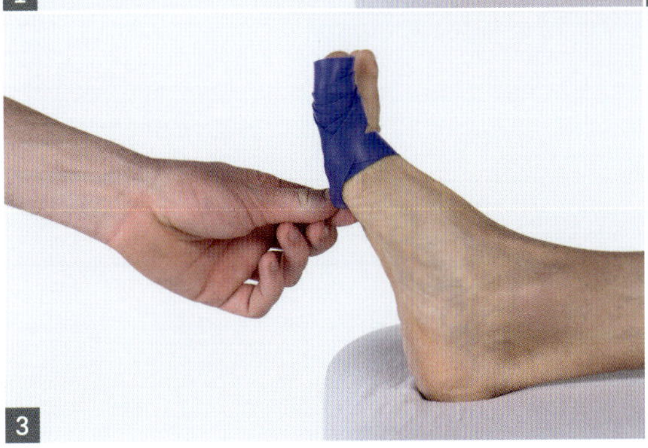

Material: Flossing band
Length: 1.03 m
Width: 2.5 cm
Tension: Medial side 60–80%, otherwise 50%

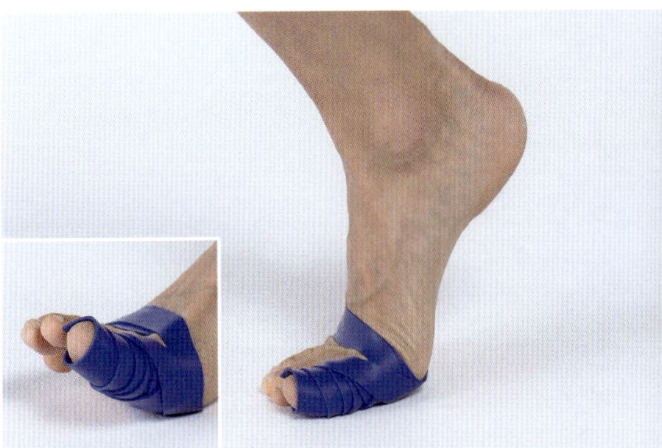

Active Exercise

Take a big step backwards, put the foot down, and extend the big toe. Or place the foot forward and push the toe up. While doing so, try to abduct it slightly. Alternatively, try to splay out the foot as far as possible or abduct the toe against gentle pressure from the outer side (press the finger lightly against the toe, the toe returns this pressure).

A Word of Advice > Hallux valgus can lead to damage to the cartilage (osteoarthritis) and should therefore be treated with conservative measures at an early stage.

Swellings of the thigh

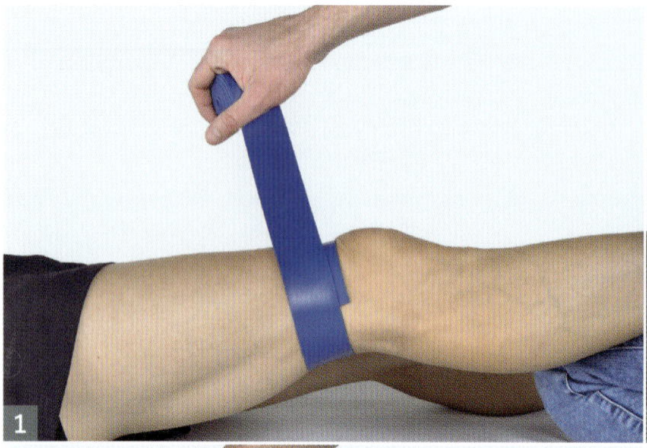

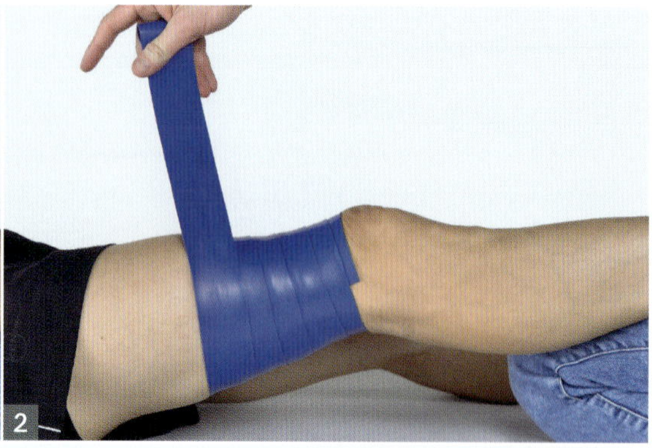

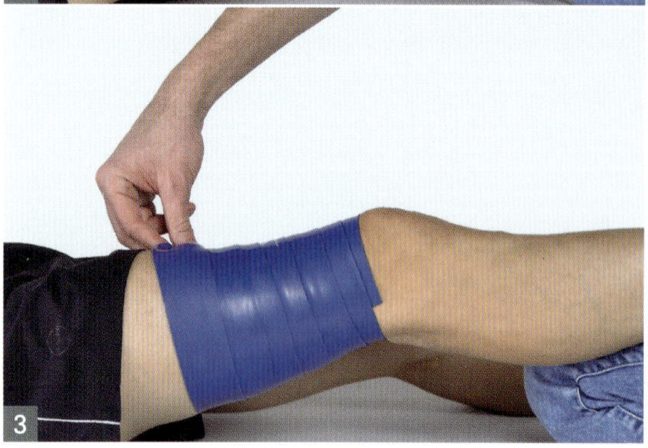

Material: Flossing band
Length: 2.06 m
Width: 5 cm
Tension: 50% overall

Swellings of the thigh

Swellings of the thigh frequently occur following a contusion or due to the action of any other direct force. A swelling indicates that the tissue fluid cannot drain away quickly enough.

The flossing band wrap
⇢ Here's how it works

1 The patient lies supine, the affected leg is raised slightly or supported. Wind the first turn with 50% tension to anchor the band below the swelling on the thigh.

2 Now wind the flossing band in ascending circular turns. The band should overlap 50% each time. A constant tension of 50% should be applied over the entire swollen region.

3 Using the same technique, wind the band upwards around the whole swelling and secure it into place.

Scars

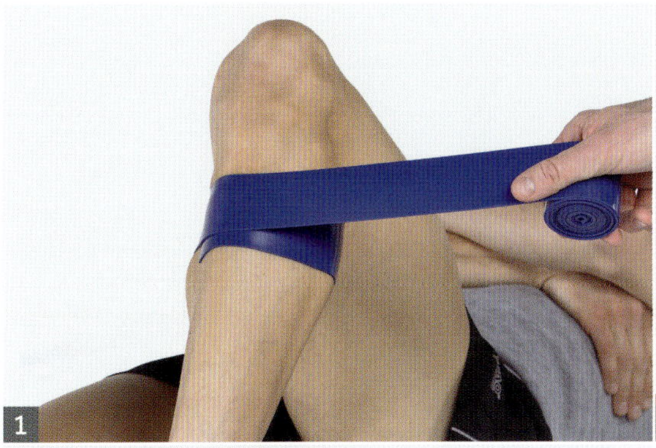

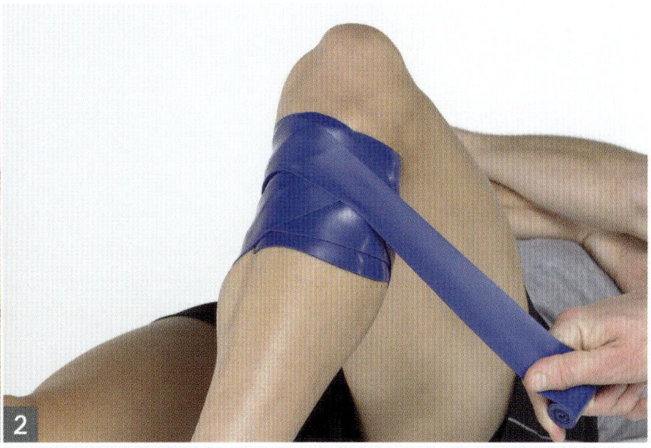

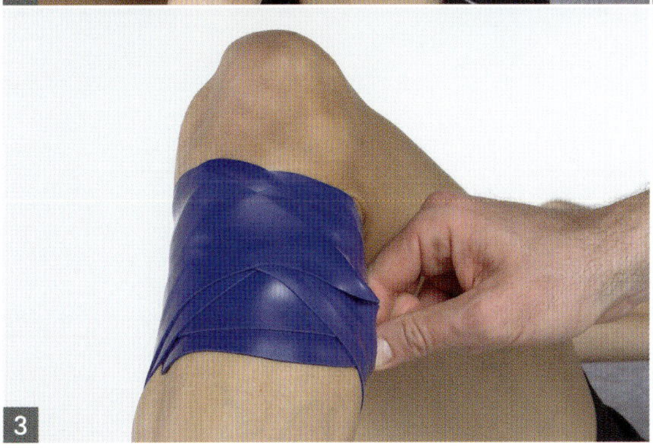

Material: Flossing band
Length: 2.06 m
Width: 5 cm
Tension: Scar 60–80%, otherwise 50%

Scars

Scars may form e.g. as a result of a surgical procedure. This involves cutting through several layers of tissue and then suturing them together again. Adhesions can form between these tissue layers, so that a joint may no longer move freely or may hurt on movement. To prevent these adhesions, the flossing band can be applied at an early stage but can also be used on old scars.

The flossing band wrap ⇢ Here's how it works

1 The affected area should be held mid-way between stretching (extension) and adduction. Wind the first turn with 50% tension to anchor the band below the scar.

2 Now wind the flossing band in ascending circular turns. The band should overlap 50% each time. A tension of 60–80% should be applied over the scar, otherwise apply a tension of 50%.

3 Using the same technique, wind the band upwards around the whole scar and secure it into place. If required, the band can also be crossed over again over the scarred area.

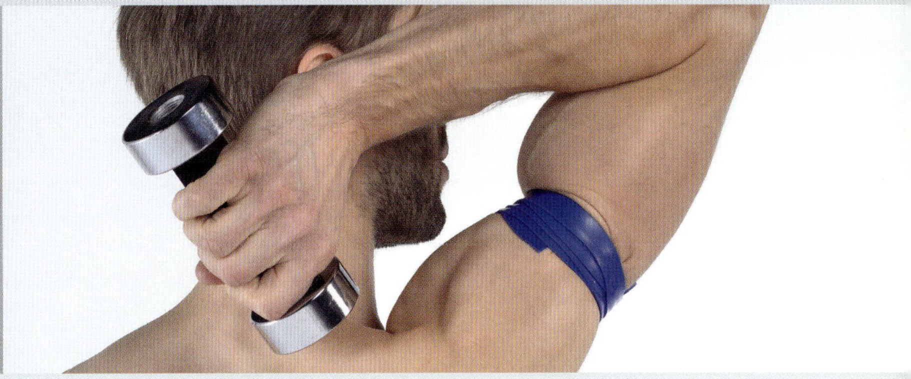

Chapter 4: Flossing Band Wraps as Strength Training

Strengthening the thigh

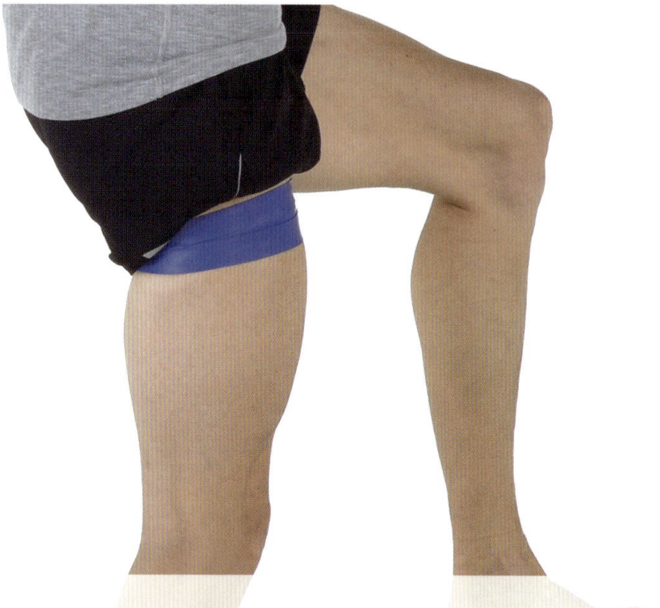

Thigh extensor (quadriceps femoris muscle)

Strengthening of the quadriceps femoris muscle is beneficial not only to athletes involved in endurance and strength sports, but also, and in particular, to patients with knee injuries. The low training intensity allows this exercise to be performed by those with osteoarthritis symptoms, during rehabilitation following knee surgery, or by elderly individuals. The quadriceps stabilizes the knee joint and works in synergy with the posterior cruciate ligament. Remember that the exercises shown here are just examples. A great variety of endurance and strength exercises can be performed with the correct Blood Flow Restriction Training wrap.

The flossing band wrap ⇢ Here's how it works

Step exercise without the wrap

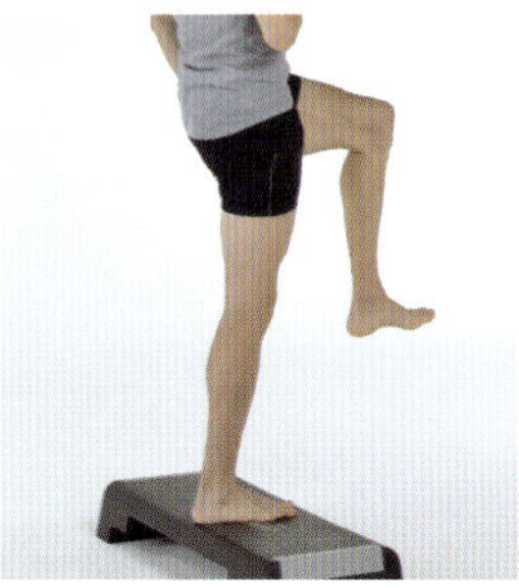

1 Apply the band to the upper third of the thigh between patella and groin. Wind it evenly and tightly enough to feel definite compression of the thigh, but without causing pain. You need to be able to tolerate the wrap for a prolonged period.

2 Place the foot on a step, a stable stool, or a bench and step up. Flex the other leg approx. 90° in the knee and hip. Do this exercise 30 times in the first set. After this, take a break (30 seconds to one minute). There should only be 15 repetitions in each subsequent set. You should do a total of 4–5 sets, with the following repetition pattern: 30-15-15-15-15.

3 Remove the band only after completing the last set. If you start to experience increasing tingling or pain during the exercise sets, take the band off immediately.

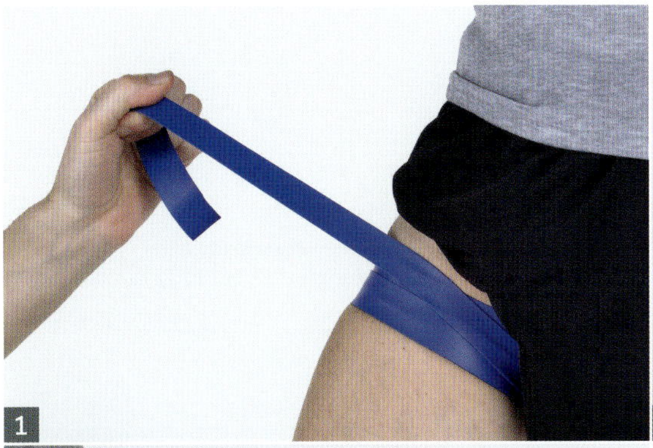
1

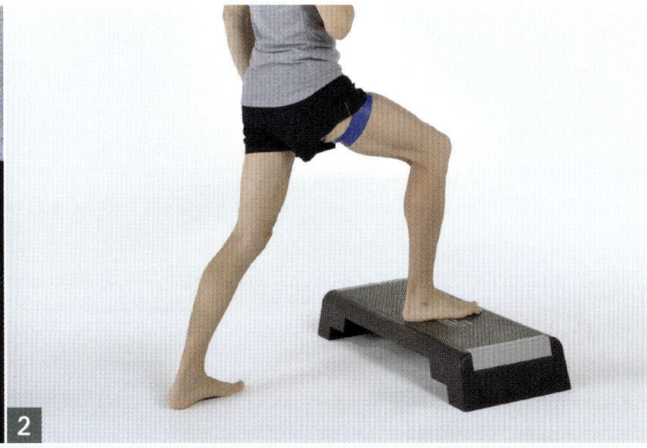
2

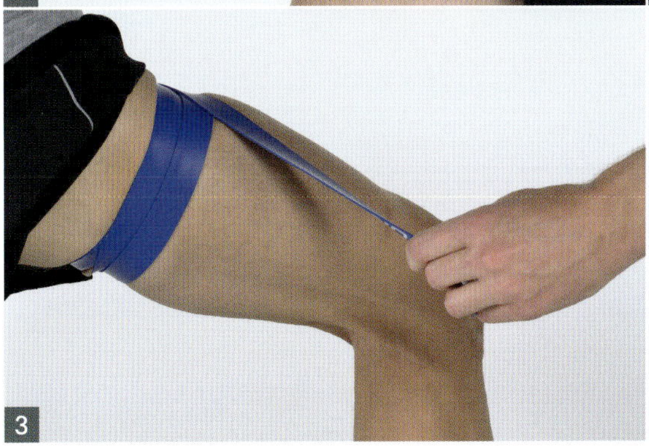
3

Material: Flossing band
Length: 1.03 m
Width: 2.5 cm
Tension: You should be able to clearly feel the tension, but without any pain.

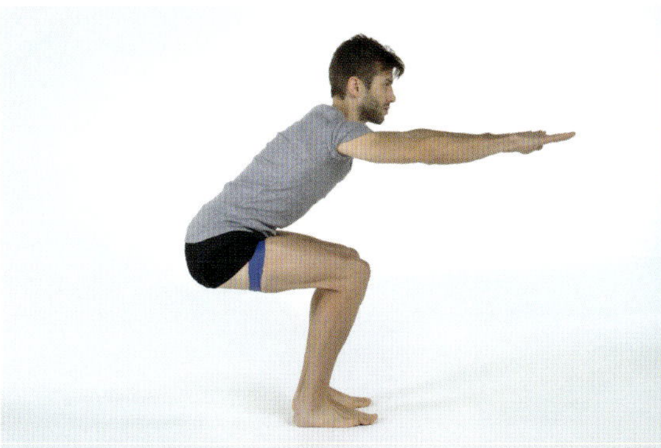

Active Exercise

After applying the band, you can perform a variety of different exercises. Once you have made sure that you follow the ground rules set out above, you can start being creative.

- Knee bends
- Lunges
- Low-resistance machine training (leg press)
- Jump-rope workout etc.

A Word of Advice > ake sure to select a step height on which you would normally be able to perform 50–70 repetitions.

Strengthening the lower leg

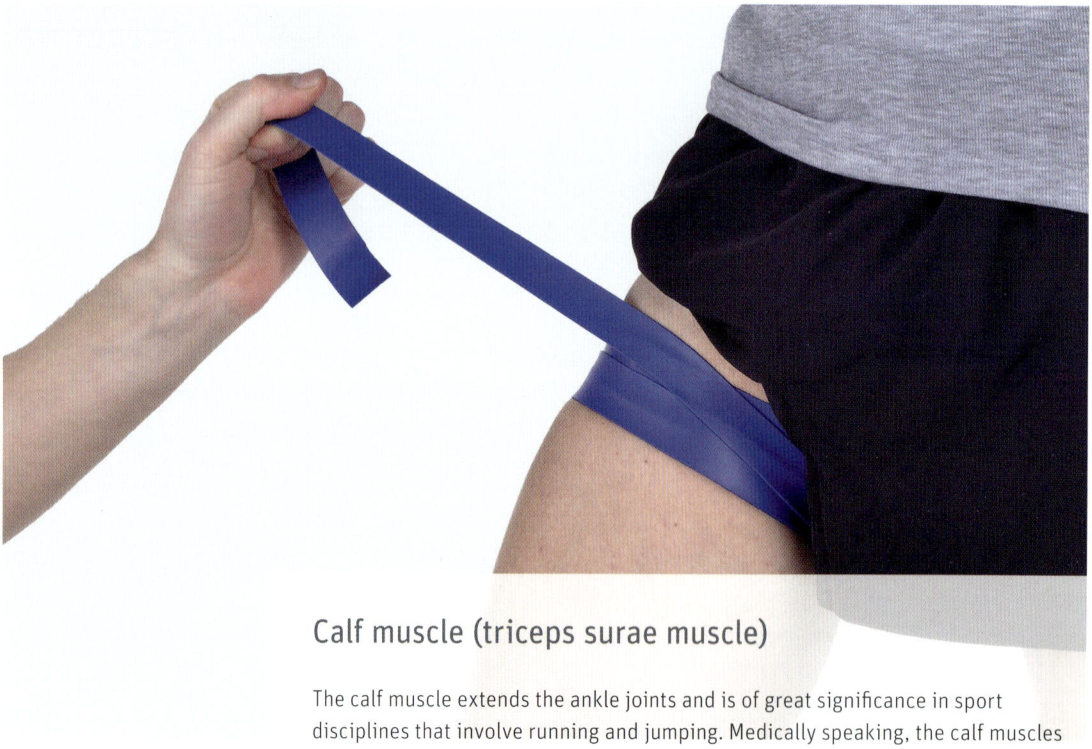

Calf muscle (triceps surae muscle)

The calf muscle extends the ankle joints and is of great significance in sport disciplines that involve running and jumping. Medically speaking, the calf muscles are relevant particularly where there is also painful inflammation of the Achilles tendon (see p. 80). Intensive eccentric training is recommended in many cases, focusing on stretching the calf muscles against resistance. The exercises are highly suitable for day-to-day use and are easy to perform.

The flossing band wrap ⇢ Here's how it works

1 Apply the band to the upper third of the thigh between patella and groin. Wind it tightly enough to feel definite compression of the thigh, but without causing pain. You need to be able to tolerate the wrap for a prolonged period.

Exercise to strengthen the calf

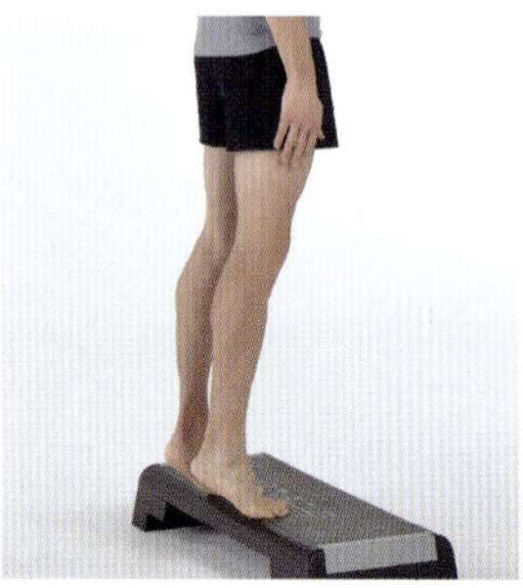

2 Stand on a step or stool on the balls of the feet. Extend both feet so that you are standing on tiptoes. Then let yourself sink down gradually. Do this exercise 30 times in the first set. After this, take a break of 30–60 seconds. There should only be 15 repetitions in each subsequent set. You should do a total of 4–5 sets. Expressed in numerical terms, the training looks like this: 30-15-15-15-15.

3 Remove the band only after completing the last set. If you start to experience increasing tingling or pain during the exercise sets, take the band off immediately.

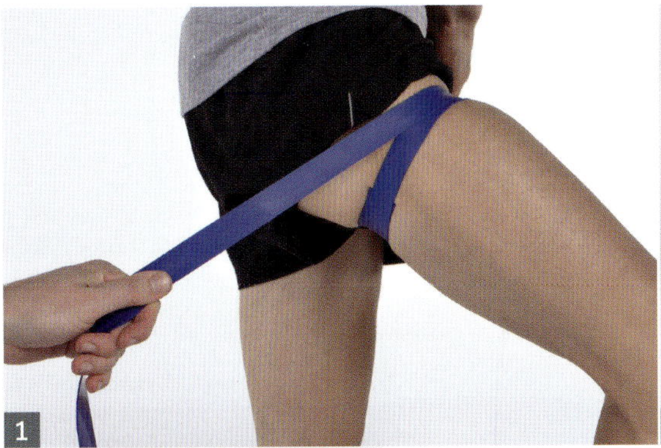

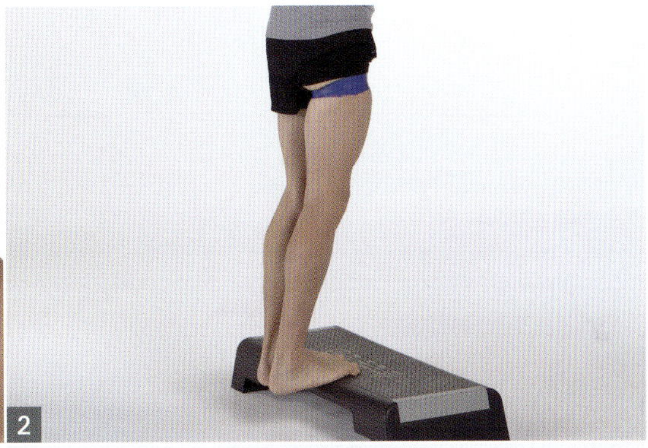

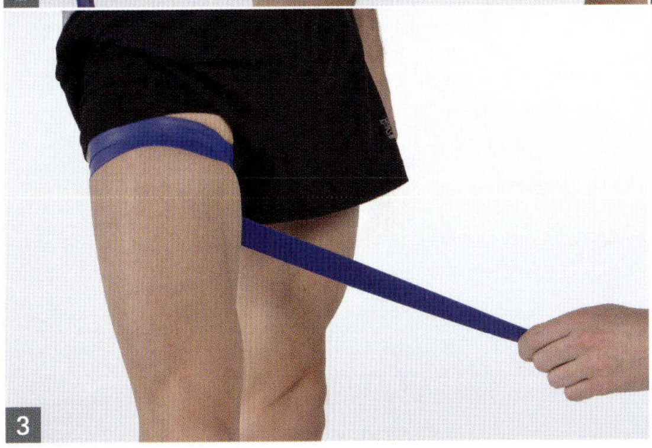

Material: Flossing band
Length: 1.03 m
Width: 2.5 cm
Tension: The tension should be high, but should not cause pain

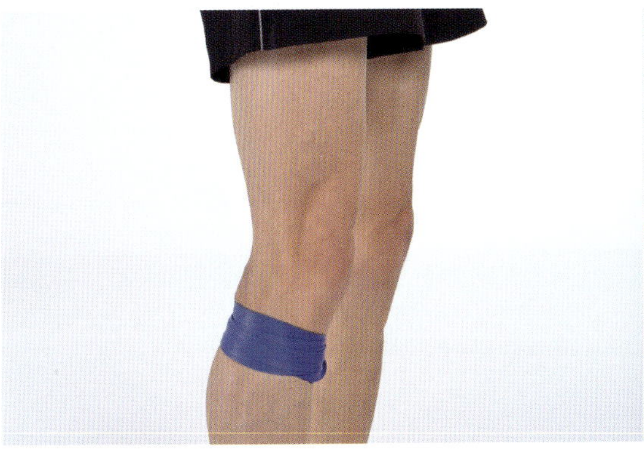

Alternative wrapping technique

As an alternative, you can also apply the bandage below the knee. By doing this, you focus on the calf muscle. In principle, however, all the leg muscles benefit from strapping the thigh.

A Word of Advice > Make sure to select a level of resistance at which you would normally be able to perform 50–70 repetitions. Do not cut off the blood supply again for at least 10 minutes after each application.

Strengthening the upper arm

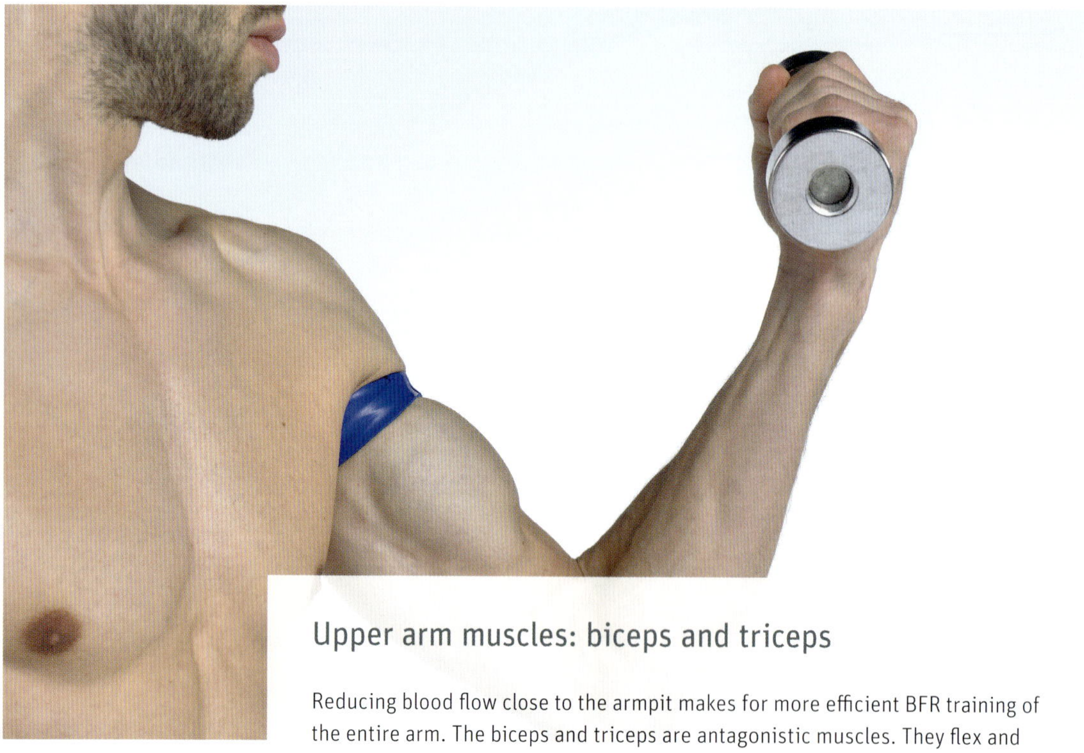

Upper arm muscles: biceps and triceps

Reducing blood flow close to the armpit makes for more efficient BFR training of the entire arm. The biceps and triceps are antagonistic muscles. They flex and extend the arm in the elbow joint and are also involved in shoulder movements. This type of training does not just benefit athletes; it can also be used to perform exercises to stabilize the shoulder or for postoperative rehabilitation.

The flossing band wrap ⇢ Here's how it works

1 Apply the band to the upper arm, as close as possible to the armpit. Wind it tightly enough to feel definite compression of the upper arm, but without causing pain. You need to be able to tolerate the wrap for a prolonged period.

2 Grasp a light weight and perform biceps flexes with it in your hand. Do this exercise 30 times in the first set. After this, take a break of 30–60 seconds. There should only be 15 repetitions in each subsequent set. You should do a total of 4–5 sets. Expressed in numerical terms, the training looks like this: 30-15-15-15-15.

3 Remove the band only after completing the last set. If you start to experience increasing tingling or pain during the exercise sets, take the band off immediately. There should be no further compression for 10 minutes after the training.

Biceps exercise, light weight

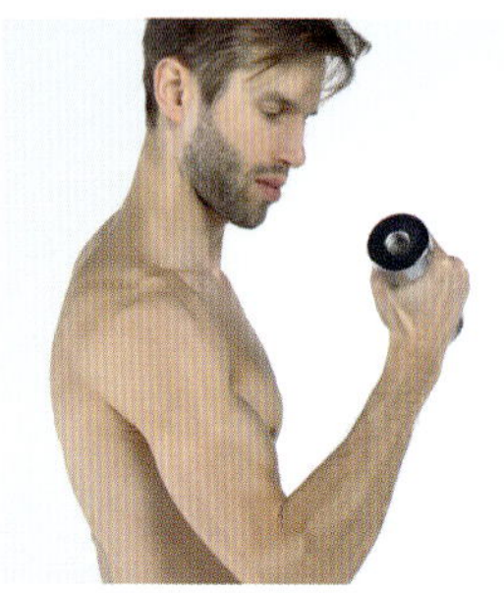

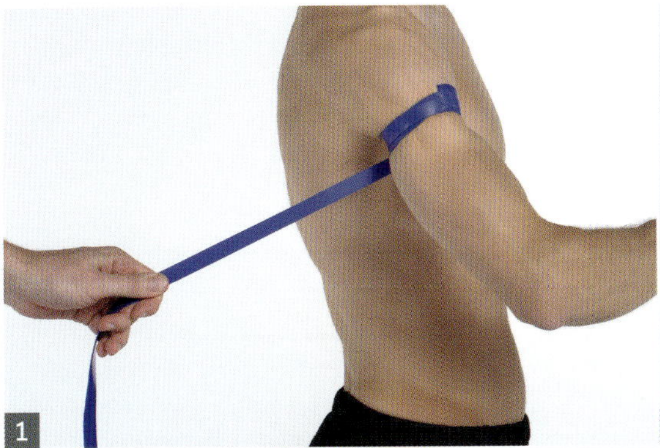

1

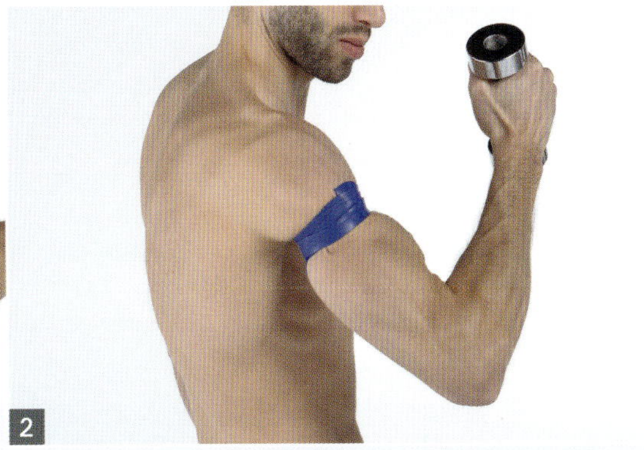

2

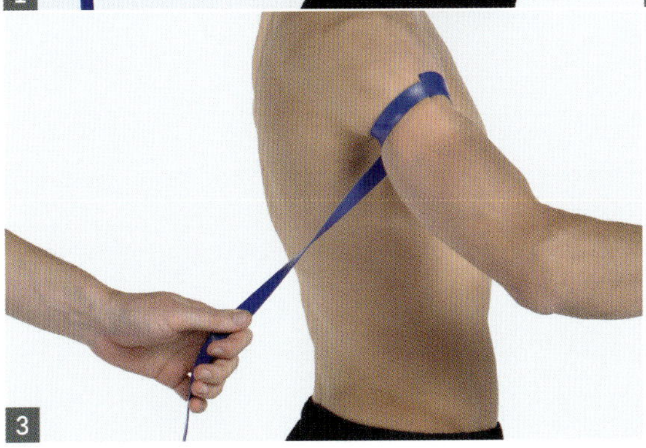

3

Material: Flossing band
Length: 1.03 m
Width: 2.5 cm
Tension: The tension should be high and uniform but should not cause pain

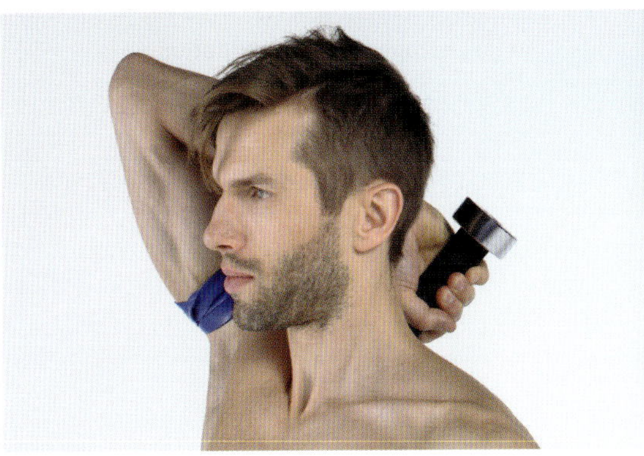

Active Exercise

Once you have absorbed and internalized the training principle, the training possibilities for the upper extremity become virtually limitless. You could perform extension exercises such as push-ups, bench pressing, and overhead extensions as well as exercises with the Thera-Band®, cable pulley, Flexi-Bar, or other training machines.

A Word of Advice > Make sure to select a level of resistance at which you would normally be able to perform 50–70 repetitions.

References

ABE T, KEARNS CF, SATO Y (2006). Muscle size and strength are increased following walk training with restricted venous blood flow from the leg muscle, Kaatsu-walk training. J Appl Physiol 100 (5): 1460–1466.

ABE T, SAKAMAKI M, FUJITA S, ET AL. (2010). Effects of low-intensity walk training with restricted leg blood flow on muscle strength and aerobic capacity in older adults. J Geriatr Phys Ther 33 (1): 34–40.

GUIMBERTEAU JC, ARMSTRONG C (2015). Architecture of Human Living Fascia. The extracellular matrix and cells revealed through endoscopy. Handspring Publishing Ltd.

HORIUCHI M, OKITA K (2012). Blood flow restricted exercise and vascular function. Int J Vasc Med: doi. 10.1155/2012/543218.

HYLDEN C, BURNS T, STINNER D, ET AL. (2015). Blood flow restriction rehabilitation for extremity weakness: a case series. J Spec Oper Med 15(1): 50–56.

OHTA H, KUROSAWA H, IKEDA H, ET AL. (2003). Low-load resistance muscular training with moderate restriction of blood flow after anterior cruciate ligament reconstruction. Acta Orthop Scand 74(1): 62–68.

SCHLEIP R (2003). Faszien und Nervensystem. Zeitschrift für Osteopathische Medizin. Volume 1/2003.

SCOTT BR, LOENNEKE JP, SLATTERY KM, ET AL. (2015). Exercise with blood flow restriction: an updated evidence-based approach for enhanced muscular development. Sports Med 45(3): 313–325.

SEIDENSPINNER D, KOLSTER BC (2015). Isokinetische und EMG-gestützte Untersuchung des Kniegelenks vor und nach einer Kompression mit einem elastischen Band. pt_Zeitschrift für Physiotherapeuten 67 (12): 52–58.

STARRETT K (2014). Werde ein geschmeidiger Leopard [Becoming a Supple Leopard]. München: Riva-Verlag.

TARADAJ J, ROSIŃCZUK J, DYMAREK R, ET AL. (2015). Comparison of efficacy of the intermittent pneumatic compression with a high- and low-pressure application in reducing the lower limbs phlebolymphedema. Ther Clin Risk Manag 11: 1545–1554.

WILSON JM, LOWERY RP, JOY JM, ET AL (2013). Practical blood flow restriction training increases acute determinants of hypertrophy without increasing indices of muscle damage. J Strength Cond Res 27(11): 3068–3075.

YASUDA T, FUJITA S, OGASAWARA R, ET AL. (2010). Effects of low-intensity bench press training with restricted arm muscle blood flow on chest muscle hypertrophy: a pilot study. Clin Physiol Funct Imaging 30(5): 338–343.

ZALESKA M, OLSZEWSKI WL, DURLIK M (2014). The effectiveness of intermittent pneumatic compression in long-term therapy of lymphedema of lower limbs. Lymphat Res Biol 12(2): 103–109.

Index